QUICK FUNCT EXERCISES FOR SENIORS

50 EXERCISES TO OPTIMIZE YOUR HEALTH

CODY SIPE, PhD

Skyhorse Publishing

Copyright © 2023 by Cody Sipe, PhD

All rights reserved. No part of this book may be reproduced in any manner without the express written consent of the publisher, except in the case of brief excerpts in critical reviews or articles. All inquiries should be addressed to Skyhorse Publishing, 307 West 36th Street, 11th Floor, New York, NY 10018.

Skyhorse Publishing books may be purchased in bulk at special discounts for sales promotion, corporate gifts, fund-raising, or educational purposes. Special editions can also be created to specifications. For details, contact the Special Sales Department, Skyhorse Publishing, 307 West 36th Street, 11th Floor, New York, NY 10018 or info@skyhorsepublishing.com.

Skyhorse® and Skyhorse Publishing® are registered trademarks of Skyhorse Publishing, Inc.®, a Delaware corporation.

Visit our website at www.skyhorsepublishing.com.

10 9 8 7 6 5 4 3 2 1

Library of Congress Cataloging-in-Publication Data is available on file.

Cover design by David Ter-Avanesyan
Cover photos by Cody Sipe, PhD

ISBN: 978-1-5107-7377-6
Ebook ISBN: 978-1-5107-7378-3

Printed in China

Contents

Introduction

At the age of 77, Minoru Saito became the oldest person to sail non-stop around the world—and he did so solo. John Glenn became the oldest astronaut and the first American to orbit the earth, at the age of 77. Yuichiro Miura summited Mount Everest at the age of 80 after previously having done so at the age of 70 and 75. Fauja Singh is credited as being the world's oldest marathon runner, having run in the Mumbai Marathon at age 104. Betty Goedhart was named the world's oldest trapeze artist, performing four to five times per year, at the age of 85 (she first tried the trapeze at the age of 78). At the age of 90, Lew Hollander became the oldest person in the world to finish an Ironman distance race which consists of a 2.4-mile swim, a 112-mile bike ride, and a 26.2-mile run. Johanna Quaas competed in gymnastics on the parallel bars into her mid-90's. And the list goes on.

What do all of these people have in common along with many, many others we could name? They didn't let their age hold them back from staying (or becoming) healthy, active, fit, and adventurous. And neither should you. Gone are the days when you can use age as an excuse to watch life from the front porch. When you could say "I'm too old to do that" and people would believe you. There are simply too many examples that would prove otherwise. From entertainers to politicians to athletes to adventurers to everyday folk—the number of older adults showing what is possible later in life is growing rapidly. And the stereotypes are beginning to fall.

This is a moment full of possibilities if you are open to them and are willing to put in the necessary time and effort to ensure that your next years are your best years. This book will enable you to create that future by optimizing your physical, mental, and functional abilities. Whether you are new to exercise or have been training a while. Whether you are somewhat fit or somewhat frail. Whether you are rather healthy or struggling with your health. The information, recommendations, and exercises you are about to learn can change your life. I know because I've worked with you before.

Over the past 30 years I have worked with older adults of all ages, ability levels, and health conditions. In fact, my career has focused almost exclusively on optimizing the health, fitness, function, and, ultimately, longevity of people over the age of 60. As a central feature of my journey, I have focused on discovering the most compelling scientific evidence from the research literature and translating that into meaningful applications. It is what led me to founding one of the most prestigious and well-respected fitness education companies in this area—the Functional Aging Institute (FAI)—and for the past 20 years, I have been able to share these evidence-based strategies with tens of thousands of fitness professionals all around the world.

The information in this book is a distillation of some of the most essential exercise principles, strategies, and exercises that have been used enhance the health, fitness, function, and longevity of thousands of people just like you. You want to significantly increase your chances of being able to keep doing all of the things you want and like to do, so don't just read the information contained here but put it into practice. You may not want to run a marathon or climb Mount Everest or be a competitive gymnast, but there are definitely some things you want to be able to do for as long as possible. What are they? Continue working. Start a new career. Travel the world. Play with your grandchildren. Take up a new hobby or sport. Live independently. Tend your garden. Hike the trails. Ski the slopes. Keep your brain sharp. Whatever it might be, I can guarantee that putting the information you are about to read into practice will help you get there.

Don't leave your future up to chance. You may get lucky and be able to stay healthy and functional without exercising, as some do, but the odds are stacked heavily against you. Think back to the past 5 or 10 years. Did your capabilities improve or worsen? Can you now do more or less? Are tasks easier or harder to do? The aging process leads us naturally toward deterioration and decay *if* we let it happen. What will your future look like if you don't make a change? What will you no longer be able to do?

What will you give up? How difficult will your life become? The single-best intervention for the negative effects of aging is exercise, and it is never too late to start reaping its benefits. Our bodies love movement, so give them what they want. Your future self will be glad you did.

Here's to your longevity,

Cody Sipe, MS, PhD, DipACLM

Chapter 1
Keys to Functional Longevity

have studied what it takes to live a long, healthy, and functional life for the past thirty years of my professional career and, along the way, I have helped many others benefit from this simple conclusion—nothing rivals the importance of eating well and moving regularly for optimal aging. Both help to drastically reduce our chances of getting chronic diseases like cardiovascular disease (the world's leading killer), type 2 diabetes, dementia (including Alzheimer's), stroke, hypertension, many forms of cancer, and osteoporosis. Either on their own are pretty powerful, but when you put the two of them together the results are even more dramatic! Would it amaze you to know that a properly designed intensive lifestyle modification program has been shown to actually *reverse* many of these conditions without the need for medications or surgeries? It is true, as it's been verified by numerous highly controlled randomized research studies.

Proper nutrition is indeed a powerful weapon against chronic disease and accelerated aging, but it cannot do for our bodies what movement can. While a balanced diet is essential for supplying all of the energy and vital nutrients our bodies require to be healthy, it is physical movement that utilizes that potential energy to grow our physical capabilities and enable us to do all of the things in life that we want to do.

Regular movement allows our bodies to grow stronger and become faster. To have greater endurance. To become coordinated and skillful. To remain resilient during times of injury and illness. To achieve higher levels of physical abilities so we can perform difficult tasks with ease. Our bodies crave movement. We were designed for it and we need a lot of it if we are to avoid the perils typically associated with growing older.

In fact, most of the physical and cognitive problems associated with getting older are not solely because people have gotten older. It's because people have not moved

1

enough and in the right ways over the course of their lifetime. Aging isn't the real problem. Inactivity is. Why are some people in their 70's, 80's, 90's, and beyond able to climb mountains, surf, run marathons, travel the world, play sports, ski, swim, and all sorts of other challenging activities? It isn't because they won the genetic lottery like many people believe. Genetics only account for about 20 percent of our health and longevity. The other 80 percent is due to our daily lifestyle choices and habits—such as how much we move and in what ways.

Our bodies are "plastic," meaning that they adapt to the challenges they are given. Stress bone, and it lays down more bone and becomes stronger. Stress muscles, and they lay down more protein to get bigger and stronger. Stress our cognitive capabilities, and they lay down new neural pathways to become more capable. This is the Principle of Adaptation at work and explains why physical movement is so important. In fact, movement is really the only way to create these kinds of beneficial adaptations. On the flip side, our bodies also adapt to a lack of movement. If our bones aren't stressed, then they lose their density and become weaker, potentially leading to osteopenia and osteoporosis. When our muscles aren't used, then they shrink and grow weaker, which can lead to frailty and disability as well as metabolic issues. So, adaptation is a two-way street which we can simply state as "use it or lose it."

Similarly, the process of aging is considered to be "plastic" as well. Although getting older is associated with a general decline in pretty much every bodily system, the good news is that the rate of decline can be modified and improved. This is because the rate of their decline is due to the simple principle of adaptation ("use it or lose it"). When you use these systems in a manner that challenges their capabilities, such as with movement, you not only improve them here and now but you actually slow down the aging process. Likewise, when you avoid movement challenges you allow the aging process to operate full-speed ahead.

This is the difference between what we might refer to as Primary (or Biological) Aging and Secondary (or Lifestyle) Aging. Primary aging occurs as part of the natural biological processes. We have been created to be born, develop/grow, reproduce, peak, decline, and eventually die. None of us will escape the ultimate end, *but* the speed at which we approach that end and the quality of our lives during the last third of life is largely up to us. And physical movement is one of the key differentiators between those who can take care of themselves and those who can't. Those who can continue to do all of the things they love to do and those who have to give them up. Those who are eager to seek new adventures and experiences and those who know they wouldn't be physically able to.

The image below represents the Functional Trajectory of Aging and highlights the range of experiences for older adults with some maintaining a high level of health and function (the blue line), while others experience a rapid decline in their health and functional ability (the yellow line). The older you get, the larger the disparity becomes. This variability is why older adults are widely considered the most heterogenous of all age groups. My experience with people on very different trajectories is what created my interest in healthy aging in the first place.

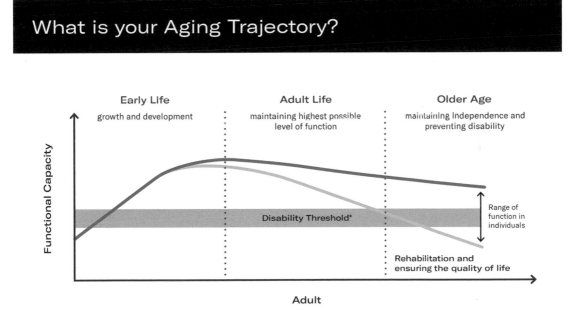

What is your Aging Trajectory?

When I was in middle school, our church youth group visited a local nursing home to sing for the residents. It was my first time going to a facility like this, and I was rather nervous since I had very little experience with older adults in general. Both of my grandfathers passed away when I was young, and I only occasionally saw my grandmothers. What stands out to me the most is the smell that hit me in the face just as I was about to enter the building. It was a weird mixture of bodily fluids and disinfectant. I actually paused at the front door and I'm not sure if I would have gone in if it weren't for my friends behind me pushing me in. As we walked to the community room, we passed by a row of residents in wheelchairs lined up in the hallways. Many were wearing what amounted to baby bibs and drooling. After our performance, we were supposed to mingle with the residents and enjoy some snacks. I stayed glued to my friends, avoiding any contact with the residents until I felt a bony hand grab my arm. I turned to find a small, frail-looking woman with white hair and (what I assumed) was no teeth. She muttered something incoherently to me and started to laugh hysterically. Frankly, the whole experience frightened me.

Fast forward to my first year in graduate school at Virginia Tech. The students helped run an exercise program for people in cardiac rehabilitation (they had previously had a heart attack or surgery). Most of them were in their 60's and 70's (with a few that were older), and based on my previous experience I was rather nervous. My fears, however, disappeared quickly, once I met the participants. They were active, relatively fit, mentally sharp, sociable, witty, and funny. Nothing like what I had experienced at the nursing home.

During my time in the program is when I realized that both experiences were valid. Some older adults are going to experience the former while others will experience the latter. Some will live out the last part of their life struggling to even take care of themselves while others will enjoy doing whatever they want to do. I decided that I wanted to help people live their best life for as long as possible—to help people in their 80's and 90's still compete in athletic events, travel the world, tackle new adventures, start new careers, and, overall, live a very high quality of life. To live the blue line life. And blue liners are popping up everywhere these days.

Growing Bolder—a multimedia company dedicated to eradicating ageist perceptions—profiles older individuals, such as athletes, musicians, actors, politicians, and artists, who are living long and well. They are the official media partner for the National Senior Games Association, which draws over 12,000 participants ages 55 to 100-plus to compete in athletic events every two years. I love to hear the stories of athletes who compete in these games. Stories like Diane Friedman who, at the age of 100, broke three masters sports records in the 100-meter dash, 200-meter dash, and javelin at the 2021 Michigan Senior Olympics in the 100 to 104 age group. People like Joe and Janet Johnston, who still compete in pole vaulting—in their 70's. They even built a 5,000-square foot pole vaulting room in their home so they could practice.

Or the story of decorated masters swimmer DeEtte Sauer (81 years old), who, ranked number one in the world in the 200-meter butterfly in her age group, didn't even start swimming until the age of 58. All of these people, and many more, are breaking the stereotypes of aging and showing how healthy, fit, and functional you can be at 70+ or even 100+.

However, you don't have to be an elite athlete to live life on the blue line.

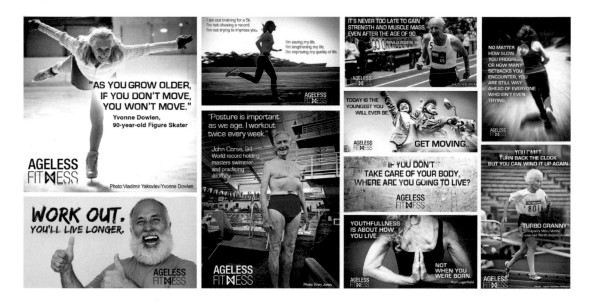

Howard is a more "real life" example of blue line living and what your 90s can look like. At the age of 92, Howard didn't look 92 and didn't fit any stereotype. He wasn't frail. He didn't seem "old" at all, except that he moved slowly and deliberately, but even then it didn't look like he was struggling at all, just that he didn't want to hurry. He was tremendously witty, and always had a joke (often dirty) to tell. Howard had given up golfing a few years back, only to find out a few years back meant as he said, "oh around age 88 or 89 I forget—and not 'cause I forget things." In fact, Howard didn't seem to forget anything. With great detail he would wax eloquently about all the sports legends from the '30s and '40s as clear as if it were yesterday.

Howard was also incredibly strong for someone in their nineties, even though by his standards all of his strength had left him. He had spent so much time in his earlier years building up so much strength that what he had left in his 90s was actually beyond that of the average 60-year- old. He also played college sports and stayed physically active through his adulthood.

His mind also stayed incredibly sharp until the very end of his life at the young age of 94. Sure, he slowed down at the end, but he still walked on his own, went out for breakfast with the boys, and outlived most of his contemporaries. He was able to do this because he had built a tremendous amount of physical reserve when he was younger so that even in his 90s he still had plenty of strength, stamina, and energy to do everything he needed to do independently.

Howard isn't a unique case. There are entire populations of people living their best life well into their 80s and 90s fully healthy and functional. These population pockets are known as blue zones, and they have been well documented by Dan Buettner in the book by the same name. In investigating what has contributed to these people's long, healthy, functional lives, researchers identified several key lifestyle factors: 1 – A predominantly plant-based diet with very little meat, dairy, or processed foods; 2 – A strong sense of purpose; 3 – Supportive relationships with family and friends; and 4 – Daily movement and lots of it.

People in the blue zones tend to live very simple but very active lives. They walk up and down hillsides; chop and carry firewood; herd livestock; plant, tend, and harvest gardens; take care of their properties; prepare their meals from scratch; and perform many other tasks week in and week out. Their bodies are not only constantly in motion, but also do chores that require a wide variety of movements such as lifting, reaching, stooping, squatting, climbing, walking, and carrying. Downtime tends to be spent with family and friends for meals and socializing rather than mindlessly watching TV or movies.

The message: If you want to live the blue line life, you will need to work for it, and the earlier you get started the better.

On the opposite end of the spectrum, there are people (too many) in their 60's and 70's who are already struggling with activities of daily living such as shopping, carrying groceries, climbing stairs, taking care of their yard, or performing their job duties. These are your yellow liners, and their futures are rather bleak. Some of the yellow line folks will end up dependent or disabled which means they are no longer able to take care of themselves and must rely on others for even simple daily tasks such as dressing, bathing, feeding, etc. Obviously, this is a worst-case scenario, but one that many people are experiencing.

The message: If you want to live the yellow line life, then don't worry about your lifestyle and just take it easy.

Of course, these two lines represent the "high" and "low" ends of the spectrum, with people falling at all points along this continuum. You may believe, as many people do, that the most important factor that determines whether you live on the blue line or the yellow line is genetics. However, this type of thinking is far from accurate. Your genes only account for about 20 percent of your health and longevity. The other 80 percent is your lifestyle. Your lifestyle has four times the impact on your future than your genes. So the Trajectory of Functional Aging actually highlights the differences between those that follow healthy lifestyles that includes lots of movement (the blue line) and those that follow unhealthy lifestyles who are sedentary or insufficiently active (the yellow line).

Howard and the Blue Zones populations are able to stay well above the dreaded disability threshold, but they are also able to stay mostly above another important threshold—the fun threshold. Crossing this point means you have to start giving up or modifying activities that you enjoy doing because they start to become too difficult. These changes may seem small at first, so small that we might not be fully aware that they are happening, but they insidiously accumulate over time. Instead of walking 18 holes of golf, you now use a golf cart. No singles tennis anymore. You now only play doubles (or give up tennis altogether for pickleball). Push-mowing the lawn has become too difficult, so now you hire someone else to do it for you. Taking carry-on luggage at the airport? Too much hassle, just check it. Take the stairs? Why don't we use the elevator instead? On and on the list goes. Changes that are seemingly innocuous at first (you're just getting older right?) become more and more impactful as the years roll on. Then, at some point, you look back at your life and ask yourself "How did I get to this point?"

So where are you on this continuum? Are you living closer to the blue line or the yellow line?

Let me pose a hypothetical scenario. Imagine that I have been bestowed with magical powers to grant you one of two wishes and the choice is yours. One, I can grant you longevity, guaranteeing that you will live a very long time. Want to live to 100? No problem. 110? Piece of cake. One hundred twenty or more? Definitely a possibility! *Or* I can grant you good health and function for however long you happen to live. You may die tomorrow, you may die next year, or you might not die for a very long time. Regardless of how long you live, however, I will guarantee that you will be able to do all of the things you need to do and like to do right up to the end. So, choice one is a guarantee of quantity with no guarantee of quality. Choice two is a guarantee of quality with no guarantee of quantity.

Which would you choose?

If you chose number two, the guarantee of quality (i.e. good health and function), then you are not alone. I have posed this question to probably thousands of people over the years and I have yet to have anyone choose longevity over function. No one wants to live a long time if it means they have to live in a care facility depending on others to take care of their basic needs or are not able to spend quality time with their family and friends. Or they're on a dozen medications and constantly having to go to the doctor. Or, maybe the worst, they're unable to even recognize or communicate with even their closest family and friends. We all realize that there is a difference between being alive and fully living. I believe that, deep down, we all desire that full, abundant life and would gladly trade in a few years if that meant a better quality of life. However, what most people don't truly understand is that they are making those choices every single day and have been for a long time.

The impact of decades of suboptimal nutrition, not enough movement, lots of sitting, stress, busyness, and many other factors typically begin to take their toll on a person in their 40's and 50's. They start to gain weight and suffer from low levels of energy. Their blood pressure and cholesterol start to creep up, oftentimes requiring medication. They begin to experience some aches and pains in their joints. More strenuous activities that they could do in their 20's and 30's are now a little too much. Moderate activities are now more strenuous. "I'm just getting older," they say. And because so many other people around them have similar experiences, they think it is normal. Then, in their 60's and 70's the rate of loss accelerates. Muscles shrink. Joints become tighter. Posture stoops. Balance worsens. Is this normal? Is it our destiny? As we have already discussed, the declines most people experience are due to a lack of movement.

Unfortunately, it is difficult for people to truly understand how powerful their movement choices can be or how great they could feel if they committed their time and energy to consistently engaging in a well-designed, progressive exercise routine. It can be a life-changer—and a future-changer! If you've been living the yellow line life for 50 to 60 years or longer, there is nothing you can do about past choices and lost opportunities, but all is not lost. Remember, the aging process is plastic just like our bodies and, although it may take a little more time and effort to make improvements compared to when we were younger, it is never too late to change your trajectory and make significant strides towards blue-line living.

One of my previous clients, Dorothy, is a great example of starting a functional exercise program, even late in life, can provide significant benefits. Dorothy was 82 years old, overweight, inactive, and with early stage Parkinson's Disease. She, like many people, never considered herself to be remotely athletic so she never even tried exercise. During the past 10 years of her life, however, she had noticed that even typical activities were becoming more difficult to do and she didn't have the energy she used to. Then came the diagnosis of Parkinson's, which would inevitably lead to a progressive deterioration of her physical abilities to the point where she would be unable to care for herself. She was the epitome of someone living life on the yellow line destined to cross the disability threshold. There was a ray of light in her rather grim future, however, and that was the opportunity to visit the Galapagos Islands with her husband. This was a dream opportunity for her. It was an opportunity, though, that she quickly realized wouldn't happen unless she got in better shape. The tour guides stated that she would need to be able to walk 1 to 2 miles at a time over uneven ground and be able to safely get in and out of a zodiac boat (a rubber boat with large inflatable sides). These were tasks she knew were too difficult for her at the time. So, she joined a functional exercise program for the very first time in her life without even being certain it was going to help. Was she too old? Was she too far gone? Would it be dangerous? Despite all of these questions, she took the leap and committed to it. Within a few weeks, her confidence started to grow and she began to realize that she actually enjoyed exercise and looked forward to the sessions. It wasn't grueling or boring or painful like she expected it to be, and she always left with a little more energy than when she walked in. Within a couple of months, she realized noticeable improvements in her ability to walk, climb stairs, and do chores without as much fatigue as she was accustomed to. Needless to say, about 6 months after beginning her very first exercise program in her late 70's, Dorothy was taking pictures of Blue-Footed Boobies (a bird) and Giant Tortoises as she walked around the islands with her husband. Quite the turnaround! Dorothy continued to exercise for many years and made significant improvements even as her disease progressed.

Take an honest look back at your lifestyle choices since you were 30 years old (we won't implicate ourselves for choices we made in our teens and twenties). How would you characterize your levels of physical activity over that time? What active pursuits have you enjoyed—walking, hiking, sports, etc.? Have you become more active, less active, or remained just as active? Are you, or have you ever been, a formal exerciser? If so, what kinds of exercises have you done and how consistently have you done them?

If you have been active and have exercised regularly, then you have potentially put yourself in the best position to enjoy the blue line life. This book will provide an opportunity for you to make some critical updates to your exercise program that will ensure that you are following an optimal plan to defy the challenges that come with getting older. Let's face it—there are some things we like to do and other things we don't like to do (even if we know we should be doing them). We fall into patterns based more on what we enjoy and, many times even, what we are good at.

There are several other potential issues that you may want to consider. Firstly, I have witnessed many individuals who have performed the same exercise routine for years, even decades, without much change or adaptation. When I was at Purdue University, I befriended a group of older men who had started a basic weightlifting program as part of a research project about 20 years earlier. While I applaud them for remaining active and exercising regularly for that length of time, the unfortunate aspect is that most were still doing the exact same things with the exact same weights. They have failed to follow the Principle of Progressive Overload, which states that as our bodies' ability to adapt to a stimulus growth will cease unless a greater stimulus is applied. Meaning, if you are able to perform 10 reps of an exercise with 20 pounds but you keep doing it session after session, your body will get stronger until 20 pounds isn't that difficult anymore. But now that 20 pounds isn't challenging, your body will stop getting stronger. Because these men didn't really understand this principle, they missed a valuable opportunity to continue improving their physical capabilities.

This also highlights another very valuable lesson—as we get older, our physical and functional needs shift, which means our exercise program needs to shift in order to continually meet those needs. Consider balance. When we are in our 30's and 40's there is very little need to incorporate any sort of specific balance training. Balance tends to be just fine, and even if a person falls they aren't very likely to get injured. Yet once we hit our 60's, balance starts to decline somewhat rapidly and that decline accelerates in our 70's. A fall is much more likely to lead to serious injuries at this stage in life. Falls are actually the number one cause of injury death; the leading cause of traumatic head injury; and the number-one cause of hip fracture in the older population. Approximately ¼ of older adults that break their hip die within a year. Point being, as our bodies change with advancing age so should our exercise program.

So, what should you be doing to optimize your ability to be fully fit and functional for the next 10, 20, or 30+ years? What is your current program potentially missing? What individual needs are not being met by your current routine? We will cover all of that in the next chapter. For now, I want you to keep an open mind and be ready to make some changes that you might not even know you need to make.

If you have been active but not a regular exerciser then you are doing a lot better than most and you have developed a good foundation to build on. What exactly is the difference though between "active" and "regular exercise"? For example, the most common form of physical activity among older adults is walking. Now you might consider this exercise, but for most people I would disagree. Why? Because most people do not walk at a sufficient intensity to get out breath, break a sweat, or get their heart rate elevated into what we would typically refer to as a "training zone". I am not saying this is a "bad" thing. On the contrary, I wish more people just walked at a moderate pace every day for 30 minutes or more, as there are many health benefits associated with walking, including an increase in longevity. However, it is a rather low-intensity stimulus so its benefits are limited since, according to the Principle of Progressive Overload, our bodies only respond to the level of challenge that we give it. So, people begin walking regularly and, at first, it may provide somewhat of a challenge, primarily because they haven't been doing much of anything, but before long the daily walk becomes easier and easier. This tells us that our bodies have adapted to the stimulus of walking, but if we do not increase the stimulus then our adaptations will plateau.

DEFINING KEY PRINCIPLES

The Principle of Adaptation states that the body continually adapts to the challenges it is given. When we were children, our bodies thrived on challenges in order to grow and develop. Without rolling, crawling, standing, walking, and other activities, our bodies would never have fully developed. It is these new challenges that stimulate growth in early life and the same is true late in life. The difference is that, when we were young we required physical stimulation to develop normally while later in life we require physical stimulation to maintain our development, regain the development we've lost, or simply prevent declines associated with aging.

The Principle of Specificity states that how a person trains determines the type of gains they make. Simply stated, "How you train is how you gain." In other words, the kinds of exercises that a person performs and how they perform them will determine the type and magnitude of results that the person sees. This principle is obvious when we consider someone who starts a walking program because they want to improve the strength of their arms. Even to the untrained eye, this doesn't make sense. Walking may be a good choice for improving cardiovascular endurance and decreasing health risk, but it has virtually no impact at all on arm strength. It is the wrong type of program for the desired results.

The Principle of Progressive Overload states that the body must continually be challenged with more difficult tasks or exercises in order for it to continue to adapt and grow. The body will adapt only to the level of challenge that you give it and will not improve any more until it is given a greater challenge. There are lots of ways to progressively overload the body such as lifting heavier weights, completing more repetitions, performing the exercise for a longer period of time (e.g. jogging for 30 minutes instead of 20), increasing the intensity, or making a movement more complex. This book uses a myriad of movements and methods to continually overload the body's systems so that you regularly make improvements.

Another reason why just walking is insufficient is because it builds cardiovascular endurance but does little to nothing for muscle strength, power, balance, coordination, etc. (factors we will discuss in more detail in the following chapters). This highlights another important principle: The Principle of Specificity. This principle simply states that your results are dependent on how you specifically stress the body which, in practical terms, means the types of activities and exercises you perform; how intensely you do them; how long; how often; etc. In other words, your arms won't get stronger unless you train them to get stronger. Your balance won't improve unless you perform exercises that challenge your balance. You won't move faster unless you try to move faster. You get the point.

This is one that I see happening all of the time as well. Having three boys that were always active in sports, I have been to many a football and basketball game. And since one of my "hobbies" is to analyze how people move (especially older adults), I have been able to observe the difficulties numerous grandparents experience navigating the bleachers, which is a real-life example of the Principle of Specificity. Many of the grandparents that I know personally are either walkers or sloggers (slow joggers), and they don't really do anything else that is active (no formal exercise or sports participation). While these individuals can typically walk for miles with ease, climbing and navigating the bleachers are sometimes a different story altogether. Some move slowly, holding onto the railing with a death grip when it is available or other people when it is not. They appear unsteady and unsure. Oftentimes, people around them physically prepare to catch them because they expect a potential fall. Some even get up and offer a hand to help them. This is likely why the lower bleachers are typically crowded primarily with older adults, with fewer and fewer as you go higher in the stands. Walking just doesn't provide the same type of challenges to navigate the bleachers with ease. That requires much more strength, balance, and, sometimes, agility. Now take that example and multiply it across the hundreds of tasks and activities you do in a week. Does walking really help with all of those? Will walking enable you to keep doing them with ease and confidence for the next 10, 20, or 30+ years? Likely not.

If you have not been regularly active at all, then the reality is that your chances of having a sharper downward trajectory in the future is significantly greater. You are likely on that yellow line and headed towards hitting that disability threshold and, even before that, the fun threshold. Depending on your age and other lifestyle factors, you may have already started to cross that fun threshold. Have you already relinquished some activities or tasks you used to do or modified them in some significant ways to make them easier to perform? Well, if nothing changes in your lifestyle, then this trend will only continue and your world will start shrinking. At what point does someone who loves to travel begin to lose their taste for it because they now see it as just too much work? They don't want to haul luggage around from the car to the airport and back again. It is now difficult getting their carry-on into an overhead bin on the plane (often relying on others to help them, which is embarrassing). Tight connections that require a hurried walk to the other end of the airport are just too tiring. Even riding on the tram that connects terminals just isn't as easy as it used to be. So, based on these and many other factors, they travel less often and only go certain places based on their perceived level of difficulty. Deep in their mind (sometime consciously and sometimes not), they know that travel itself hasn't become more difficult but, rather, their physical abilities have decreased. The common belief is that this is because they have gotten older, although aging isn't the main problem—it's lifestyle. So, if you haven't been active, now is the time to get active, alter the trajectory you are on, and change your future for the better.

One of the primary reasons why getting and staying in great shape is important to your future is due to something called physiologic reserve. Without physiologic reserve, you are at severe risk of debilitation. You can think of this as how much ability you have left in the tank when you are performing tasks. For example, both an average person and an elite endurance athlete can walk at a brisk pace without much difficulty. However, if they had to, the elite athlete could run fast for a very long distance while the average person would have to quit after only a short distance. This is because the athlete has more in the tank that they could give if they needed to. In essence, they have greater physiologic reserve. Having greater reserves means that when you are injured or become ill, you have a much greater chance of coming out the other side without major problems. You can also recover faster and more fully.

Consider what happens to robust and healthy individuals compared to frail individuals when some stressor, like an illness or injury, comes along. The robust person takes a temporary hit on their functional abilities, but they bounce back quickly and return to their previous levels. A pre-frail or frail person, however, doesn't fully recover.

OPTIMIZING BRAIN HEALTH AND FUNCTION

So far, we have focused on physical abilities but not nearly as much on cognitive abilities. Study after study shows that physical activity, diet, and other lifestyle factors keep the brain healthy as we age—contrary to the popular notion that cognitive function inevitably declines in the later years of life. Admittedly, Alzheimer's disease and other dementias pose serious health risks. Alzheimer's is one of the leading causes of death for Americans over 65, and the threat keeps rising: In the next decades, the number of cases worldwide is expected to nearly triple, from 46.8 million in 2015 to 131.5 million in 2050 (Alzheimer's Association 2017; ADI 2015). And another 15 to 20 percent of older adults are diagnosed with mild cognitive impairment (MCI), according to the Alzheimer's Association. But this doesn't mean brain power must wane as we age. Research overwhelmingly suggests that cognitive function in old age reflects how people live: Nutrition, stress, environment, physical activity, relationships, and even individual views on aging play a role. And recent advances in neuroscience suggest that aging adults retain the ability to improve their neural networks and cognitive function—a concept scientists call neuroplasticity.

Dementia is an umbrella term for multiple cognitive impairments whose symptoms include memory loss, poor judgment, communication difficulties, and personality changes. Alzheimer's disease, the most common cause of dementia, has several risk factors, including age, family history, and genetics. While several genes are known to increase the risk of Alzheimer's, many people with these genes do not develop the disease. Hence, it stands to reason that other important risk factors—either disease or lifestyle-related—play a role.

Cardiovascular and metabolic conditions such as heart disease, type 2 diabetes, hypertension, high blood cholesterol levels, and obesity significantly increase a person's chances of developing dementia. In fact, cardiovascular disease or diabetes doubles the risk (Alzheimer's Society 2016). Other conditions, such as kidney disease, anxiety, and sleep apnea, have been linked to dementia in some studies, but the evidence is still weak.

There is overwhelming evidence that certain lifestyle factors play a significant role in dementia risk just as they do with almost all other chronic conditions. Most of these factors are also closely linked to the risk of cardiovascular disease, so it could be said that "what is good for your heart is also good for your head." The three primary lifestyle risk factors are physical inactivity, smoking, and an unhealthy diet.

The good news is that our brains respond to stimuli just like our bodies do. Many perceive their brains as a computer, which is not too far off, only it is a living computer. Just as a computer depends on hardware and software to operate, so do our brains. The hardware is the brain as an organ. And like any other organ, it depends on good blood flow, oxygenation, and nutrients. This is why some chronic disease conditions, such as cardiovascular disease, are closely linked to brain health. Just as the heart can develop plaques in its arteries which may build up to the point of impairing blood flow, so can other organs such as the brain. Brain cells (neurons) are like plants that depend on rich soil in order to grow, be healthy, and produce. Without that rich soil, the neurons do not propagate more neurons.

The software is the neural circuitry that serves as the brain's operating system and allows it to "think." The number of neurons (brain cells) is an important factor, but how they are integrated to the neural network is another. Just having a lot of neurons isn't enough. They need to be connected to other neurons in a purposeful manner in order to assist with cognition.

To optimize brain function, you need to understand the variety of cognitive tasks we perform daily, such as reasoning, memory, attention, language, and physical movement. These play key roles in our lives, but arguably the most important cognitive task is executive function—encompassing the higher-level skills that control and coordinate other cognitive abilities.

Executive function is loosely divided into organizational and regulatory abilities:

- Organization includes attention, planning, problem-solving, working memory, cognitive flexibility, and abstract thinking.
- Regulation includes self-control, initiation of action, emotional regulation, inhibitory control, moral reasoning, and decision-making.

Cognitive decline usually affects specific aspects of executive function. For example, people with MCI may have significant memory loss (forgetting important information they would previously have recalled with ease, such as appointments, conversations, or recent events), while others may lose thinking skills (ability to make sound decisions or to judge the time or sequence of steps needed to complete a complex task). Typically, memory impairments happen first. A decline in thinking skills may indicate a progression toward dementia. While those with MCI are at greater risk of developing Alzheimer's disease, they don't always get it. In some cases, MCI reverts to normal cognition, according to the Alzheimer's Association.

In order to retain excellent cognition as we get older, it is important to keep both the hardware and software sides of our brains healthy and functional. There are three key processes that are important to consider—angiogenesis, neurogenesis, and synaptogenesis. Angiogenesis is the stimulation of new blood vessel growth in the brain, which increases its oxygen and nutrient supply. Neurogenesis is the stimulation of new brain cells. Contrary to popular belief, you *can* teach an old dog new tricks and you can create new brain cells at any age. Synaptogenesis is the creation of new connections between brain cells as they become integrated into the larger neural network of the brain. This is the ultimate end result that we are seeking in order to optimize brain function. These three key processes demonstrate a dynamic continuum between the hardware side of the brain and the software side of the brain. It also should provide some clues as to what kinds of activities and challenges are going to optimize brain health and cognitive function over the course of a lifetime. And at the core is movement.

Your brain loves movement. It thrives on it. Two forms of movement that have a significant impact on the hardware side of the brain are cardiovascular exercise and strength training. These two forms of movement stimulate blood flow to the brain and the production of beneficial neurotrophic factors, which are both critical to maintaining good brain health and function.

NEUROPLASTICITY

The ability of the brain to form and reorganize synaptic connections, especially in response to learning or experience or following injury.

The brain's ability to adapt both structure and function throughout life and in response to experience.

ANGIOGENESIS

The development of new blood vessels, which helps to increase the flow of oxygen and nutrients to cells.

NEUROGENESIS

The process by which new neurons (brain cells) are formed in the brain, which is stimulated by physical and cognitive activity.

SYNAPTOGENESIS

The formation of synapses, the points of contact where information is transmitted between neurons, which is integral for creating brain networks.

Aerobic exercise and resistance training are good for the brain. If frequency and intensity are sufficient, either of these can have a significant impact on brain function. And when you do both of them, the results are typically even better (Bamidis et al. 2014; Hotting & Roder 2013; Szuhany, Bugatti & Otto 2015). While there are some similarities in how these two forms of exercise help the brain, there are also some unique differences.

Cardiovascular fitness is closely associated with cognitive health with advancing age. Higher levels of cardiovascular fitness are generally associated with higher levels of cognitive function plus better brain size and structure in cross-sectional studies of older adults. Improved brain blood flow is one of the benefits of cardiovascular exercise, but research suggests that stimulation of a protein called brain-derived neurotrophic factor (BDNF) is a key mechanism for cognitive improvements after aerobic exercise training. You may have heard of BDNF, as it is considered so important for brain growth that it has been dubbed "Miracle Gro for the Brain." It plays an especially vital role in the development of new nerve tissues (i.e. neurogenesis) and, yes, contrary to popular belief, older adults can still grow new brain cells. Higher levels of BDNF are associated with better spatial, episodic, and verbal memory, while lower levels of BDNF—particularly in older adults—have been linked to atrophy of the hippocampus and may contribute to memory impairment (Szuhany, Bugatti & Otto 2015). The great news is that BDNF levels can increase after just a single session of aerobic exercise. You could go out for a moderate 30-minute walk right now and immediately the BDNF levels in your brain will rise. What's more is that they will rise even more with regular exercise. How much do you need? Just 30-plus minutes of moderate-intensity movement, enough to elevate your heart rate and increase your breathing rate, 5 days per week is sufficient…but of course, more may be even better.

Regular resistance exercise (e.g. strength training or weight lifting) has also been shown to improve cognitive function, although this type of training has been studied far less than aerobic exercise. The research suggests that resistance exercise may stimulate cognition by increasing levels of insulin like growth factor 1 (IGF-1). Since BDNF and IGF-1 are thought to collectively stimulate the three key processes for brain growth—neurogenesis, synaptogenesis (formation of new synapses), and angiogenesis (formation of new blood cells)—through interacting pathways, the combination of aerobic and resistance training can potentially provide even greater results. Two to three days per week of 20 to 30 minutes of weight lifting is all it takes…but, once again, more may be even better.

There are other variables to also consider which may further enhance your results. Working out in group settings potentially provides more social stimulation than exercising independently. Social interaction has been identified as an important factor in brain health so it is possible that exercising with others may be better. Outdoor exercise may provide greater sensory stimulation than exercising indoors. Hiking, for example, requires better navigation and coordination skills and provides a much higher level of sensory stimulation compared to walking on a treadmill which, again, may be better.

If you simply performed aerobic exercise five days per week and strength training two days per week, you would likely improve your brain health and fitness significantly. However, the most effective strategy for boosting brain health is likely to be a combination of physical exercise with cognitive challenges in a rich sensorimotor environment. Let me break down what this means exactly starting with the combination of physical and cognitive tasks. For one, this does not mean trying to do a Sudoku puzzle while walking on the treadmill. While this "dual task" strategy is technically a way to combine a physical task with a cognitive task, there is evidence that the cognitive challenges should be linked directly to the physical tasks that are being performed. For example, when a person plays pickleball, they have to quickly think through where they want to play the ball in specific situations according to their opponent's abilities while they are constantly moving around the court and hitting the ball. Almost all sports, in fact, require this combination of physical and cognitive challenges. They also provide the additional element of being in a rich sensorimotor environment. All that means, really, is that the individual is having to use their five senses to be aware of, and interact with, elements in their environment. Other types of activities, such as tai chi, dance, and "exergames" also provide all of these elements and have documented benefits for brain health (Bamidis et al. 2014). Each of these activities requires constantly planning, scaling, anticipating, adjusting, responding to, and coordinating movements to accomplish a task, which keeps the brain fully engaged with the body.

Lastly, a simple way to ramp up your brain power is to try something new. Learning a new physical skill is a powerful way to stimulate those neurons since the brain is what controls all physical movement. Ever try to brush your teeth with your non-dominant hand? It feels awkward and unnatural and you will probably end up brushing most of your face. But what if you used that hand to brush your teeth every day for the next three months? Would you get better at it? Would it start to feel more natural? Of course it would, because your brain would learn how to perform those fine movements with that hand and the learning process is what will enhance your brain's functioning. So pick up a new musical instrument or try out a new sport or learn how to juggle or, if you dare, start brushing your teeth with your off hand. Whatever you choose to do will help to enhance your brain's abilities.

PHYSICAL-COGNITIVE EXERCISES FOR BRAIN HEALTH

Sports: If you already enjoy playing a sport, especially one that requires cardiovascular endurance such as tennis, pickleball, racquetball, volleyball, basketball, or soccer, then you are already well on your way to optimizing your brain function, so don't stop. In fact, you should consider picking up a new sport—one that you used to do or one that you've never tried before. The novelty of the sport will require a much higher demand on motor learning, thus increasing the cognitive challenge which should provide an even greater stimulus to brain growth. And if you haven't been playing a sport at all, then get out there and try a few until you find one that you really enjoy. Be sure to choose something that meets your current level of physical and cognitive abilities so that you don't get too frustrated.

Dance: Do you know what kind of dance is the most cognitively stimulating? Line dancing? Salsa? Ballroom? It could be any of these or it could be none of these, because it is actually the dance that you don't know how to do yet. The novelty or difficulty of the dance is what provides the cognitive stimulation. So, if you have been line dancing for decades and know those moves "by heart," then it has lost some of its cognitive stimulation. Your brain has already learned it and it is time to try something new. You could learn a brand-new line dance routine or try a different genre altogether. The different beats, rhythms, speed, flow, and movement styles could provide a different level of cognitive stimulation altogether. For the non-dancers out there—it will all be new, so just pick something that looks fun.

Tai Chi: This ancient form of martial arts is often referred to as "movement meditation," and it is one of the most well-studied forms of specialized exercise for older adults. Its benefits for health, function (especially balance), and cognition are widely documented. There are different styles of Tai Chi that are taught but throughout all of them the movements require weight shifting, stepping in multiple directions, turning, bending, and coordinating arm movement patterns. Once you learn the basic forms you put them together into a flow (sequence). After that you could spend the rest of your life trying to perfect your precision, control and breathing which makes it perfect for beginners as well as the most experienced.

BRAIN GAMES

Brain-training programs and games have blossomed into a competitive industry with direct consumer spending on digital brain-health software products expected to reach $1.52 billion by 2020 (Simons et al. 2016). Companies such as Lumosity, Posit Science, Cogmed, and CogniFit advertise the brain-boosting benefits of their software platforms. But do these products really work? The scientific evidence is somewhat scattered, but several recent reports (Simons et al. 2016) conclude that brain-training games do not reduce the risk of cognitive decline or dementia. They can significantly improve specific cognitive processes—but not much else.

LIMITS OF BRAIN TRAINING

So, what about all of those "brain training" apps and games? Are they worth the time and effort? The answer is a resounding: maybe. The saying that "doing crossword puzzles only makes you better at doing crossword puzzles" is somewhat true. Indeed, the U.S. Federal Trade Commission charged a large brain software company with "deceptive advertising" because it could not produce sufficient data supporting its claims on the efficacy of its games (Peterson & Fung 2016). Research on computerized brain training demonstrates that the benefits are limited to whatever brain processes are used by the game but that the other cognitive functions remain much the same (Ballesteros et al. 2015). For example, an intervention challenging verbal working memory improves that skill. However, neither closely related skills, such as spatial working memory, or more distant skills are affected.

Probably the strongest evidence of cognitive training's effectiveness emerged from the ACTIVE study (Ball et al. 2002), which is the most rigorous, comprehensive trial to date. Over 2,800 older subjects were randomly assigned to one of three cognitive interventions (memory, speed of processing, and reasoning) or a no-contact control group. Participants completed 10 sessions over a period of 5 to 6 weeks, with some receiving four booster training sessions a year later. The study showed that the trained skills improved, but it found no transfer to other skills. Improvements lasted up to 2 years after training.

THE BOTTOM LINE

Regularly performing cognitively-stimulating activities, such as software games, crossword puzzles, or board games (e.g. chess), are beneficial for stimulating specific aspects of brain function, and would certainly be a better choice for your leisure time compared to non-stimulating activities, but they should not be relied upon solely to optimize your brain health and cognition as you age.

BRAIN EXERCISE PROGRAMS

The cognitive benefits of aerobic and resistance exercise depend on the FITT model of exercise prescription: Frequency, Intensity, Time, and Type. For those without any signs of cognitive decline, it is important to meet the basic recommendations for each of these, but exceeding these guidelines could potentially yield even greater benefit. For those with cognitive decline, meeting these guidelines will be helpful, but you may need to consult with a health professional in order to get a more targeted lifestyle prescription.

The guidelines for aerobic and resistance exercise for cognition really don't differ significantly from the general recommendations for older adults for physical health and function. Perform 30 minutes or more of aerobic exercise at 60 to 75 percent of maximal heart rate on 5 or more days per week. It doesn't matter what type of aerobic exercise you choose—walking/jogging, swimming, biking, elliptical trainer, etc. The guidelines for resistance exercise are to perform 1 to 3 sets of 8 to 12 repetitions of muscle-building exercises (e.g. weight lifting) for all of the major muscle groups (8 to 10) on 2 to 3 days per week. The equipment you use (dumbbells, barbells, kettlebells, bands, bodyweight, machines, etc.) doesn't seem to matter. In the coming chapters you will learn more about the different types of movements and programming that would help meet these guidelines.

Yet how do you factor in more cognitive-physical activities such as sports or dance? Do you need to do those in addition to your aerobic and resistance exercise routines? Not necessarily. If these activities have a sufficient aerobic and/or strength component to them then, from a cognitive health perspective, they are sufficient. Plus, cognitive-physical activities are less dependent on physical intensity (e.g. heart rate) and more dependent on cognitive intensity (i.e. complexity). When you are learning a new dance step, for example, it isn't very likely that you will be able to perform it well enough to get your heart rate up and keep it there because in order to learn the dance you will need to slow down and practice the individual steps. Then, as you learn the steps, you will gradually be able to speed up your movements and string more steps together into longer and longer sequences until you finally know the entire dance. From this point on, the cognitive challenge will begin to decline while the aerobic challenge gradually increases. Some activities, such as tennis, may require a higher aerobic demand right from the start because your inability to hit the ball well will likely mean you have to move around quite a bit chasing the ball!

The bottom line, when it comes to optimizing your cognitive trajectory, is that you want to move a lot and your movements should include a combination of aerobic, resistance, and cognitive-physical activities on a regular basis. Make these activities social and fun by doing them with others and you have a great recipe for success.

MINDSET: THE X FACTOR

There is another critical factor for longevity that may be even more important than movement or nutrition. It is your attitude towards aging and, more specifically, how well, or poorly, you believe you will age. The mind is a powerful tool and its connection to our physical selves is a mystery still being unraveled, but the association between our longevity and our mindset is undeniable.

In essence, those with a positive mindset about the aging process live up to seven years longer than those with a negative mindset. They tend to live healthier, happier lives as well. This phenomenon has been referred to as a self-fulfilling prophecy. Those that buy in to the negative stereotypes of aging tend to become those stereotypes—ones that communicate that to be old is to be sick, weak, poor, fragile, alone, and depressed. That older adults should retire since they can no longer contribute to their professions adequately. That they are destined to lose their independence, and even worse their minds, and live in a care home. These are just a few of the numerous stereotypes that are unfortunately all around us as they are embedded into many facets of our society that still tends to revere youth above all else. It has been stated that ageism is a prejudice toward our future selves. After all, don't we all want to live to a "ripe old age"? So, then why do so many view old age so negatively? From greeting cards to TV shows to movies to advertisements, negative images are all around us, so it's no wonder so many people believe them.

But they also believe these stereotypes because they typically know people who *are* the stereotype without fully understanding *why* they are the stereotype or giving just as much credence to those who *defy* the stereotypes. And, probably also because until recently there were a lot more stereotypes than not.

COMMON MYTHS ABOUT AGING FROM *SUCCESSFUL AGING*

Myth: To be old is to be sick.
Fact: Old age can be a healthy, vibrant, productive, and enjoyable period of life, as many people are now demonstrating. How well we age depends much less on aging, per se, and more on lifestyle. Live a healthy lifestyle that includes physical activity

and exercise and you considerably increase your odds of living longer and, maybe more importantly, better.

Myth: You can't teach an old dog new tricks.

Fact: The pervasive belief older individuals cannot sharpen or broaden their minds is disturbing. The latest research in brain aging demonstrates that the brains of older individuals still retain their neuroplasticity. They just need to be given the proper types and amounts of stimuli, like physical and cognitive challenges.

Myth: The horse is out of the barn.

Fact: Is it ever too late to recover from a lifetime of unhealthy choices? According to extensive research, it is almost never too late to begin healthy habits or benefit from those changes—many of which occur very rapidly. For example, the risk of heart disease begins to fall almost as soon as you quit smoking—no matter how long you've smoked.

Myth: The secret to successful aging is to choose your parents wisely.

Fact: The impact of genetics in aging is wildly exaggerated and only actually accounts for 20 to 25 percent of a person's longevity. The most profound effects on the aging process come from lifestyle. Healthy lifestyles literally slow down the biological processes of aging, while unhealthy choices accelerate them.

Myth: The lights may be on, but the voltage is low.

Fact: This myth suggests that older people suffer from inadequate physical, mental, and sexual abilities. Sexual activity does tend to decrease in old age but there is huge variability among individuals. The vast majority of older adults retain their desire for intimate and sexual connection.

Myth: The elderly don't pull their own weight.

Fact: If you are retired, and don't work, then obviously you are a burden to society, right? Wrong. For one, many older adults choose to keep working and even starting new businesses. Plus, they are the largest volunteer force and make up the majority of childcare in the US.

Adapted from the book Successful Aging (Pantheon 1998).

  On the other hand, there are those who view the aging process as a time of possibilities, an opportunity for growth and new experiences. A time to enjoy the benefits of a lifetime of experience. To spend more time with family. To spoil grandkids.

To try new things. To read new books. To visit new places. Those who see those elite senior athletes and are inspired by how fit, healthy, and functional they are, and it gives them hope for their own future. They don't deny that they are getting older. They see the gray hairs and wrinkles. They know they aren't as "youthful" as they used to be, but their hope for the future is bright despite these changes.

What is interesting is that most older adults report that they are now in their best stage of life and realize that many of the fears and beliefs they had about getting older when they were younger were inaccurate. Surveys of younger and middle-aged adults demonstrate that their perceptions about what older adulthood will be like don't match reality. They errantly believe that the "problems" of old age are much more common than they actually are, ranging from physical problems to cognitive issues to the revocation of driving privileges. Most of the fears about getting older are unfounded.

The message: Don't believe the negative stereotypes about getting older that are all around you. Focus on positive images, messages, and examples of how great this stage of life can be and then make choices to make them a reality for your own life.

While I'm no genie and I can't guarantee that you will live a high quality of life—fully healthy, fit, and functional—for as long as you live, I can definitely help you increase your chances significantly if you put the principles, strategies, and movements into practice that you will find in this book. So, let's go for it!

CHAPTER 2
Functional Training

I f there is one word to describe the older adult population, it is "heterogenous." An individual's chronological age is only a rough guideline as to their functional age (i.e. their capabilities), and this varies widely from person to person. Like they say in geriatric medicine, "If you've seen one 70-year-old, you've seen one 70-year-old." Although functional capacity generally decreases with advancing age, the degree and rate of decline are highly variable so that individuals of the same age can exhibit highly variable levels of function. We probably all know an 80-year-old who can physically or mentally outperform many others 10 or 20 years their younger. I know of an 80-year-old doing CrossFit who can complete workouts I wouldn't even want to try.

The physical capabilities of an individual are dependent on a wide variety of factors that have a complex relationship with one another. Consider the Six Domains of Function model below (Source: Functional Aging Institute). This is but one way to obtain a fuller understanding of what is meant when we refer to a person's functional abilities. The image below displays six primary categories (domains) that are critical to being able to function well as we age. They are: Neuromuscular; Musculoskeletal; Cardiorespiratory; Balance; Mobility; and Cognitive/Emotional. Each of these domains can be further divided into subcategories, which help to show the "behind the scenes" complexity to our human physiology.

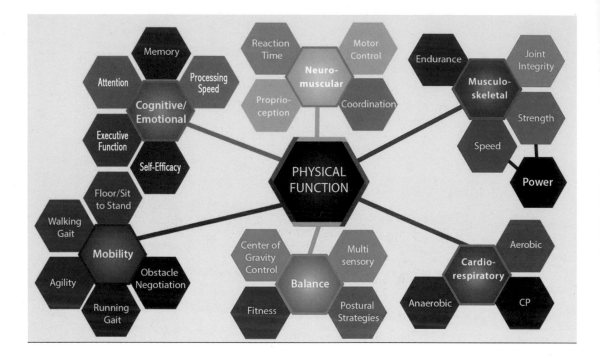

SIX DOMAINS OF FUNCTION

NEUROMUSCULAR
The ability to move in a coordinated and skillful manner. It includes factors such as motor control (turning muscles on and off with precision timing), coordination, proprioception (receptors in our joints and muscles that tell the brain about body movement), and reaction time.

MUSCULOSKELETAL
The ability of the joints and muscles to function properly. It includes how much force our muscles can create (strength); how quickly they can contract (speed and power); how long they can keep working before fatiguing (endurance); and how stable our joints are (joint integrity).

CARDIORESPIRATORY

The ability to perform continuous large-muscle movements, like walking, swimming, or biking. This is dependent on the conditioning of the cardiovascular system and peripheral factors (like mitochondria). It includes very short-burst movements like running a few steps quickly to jump over a puddle; short distance high-intensity activities (anaerobic) like a sprint; and longer duration (aerobic) activities like jogging a mile.

BALANCE

The ability to avoid falling by controlling your center of gravity over your base of support. It is a complex system of sensory input (especially vision, somatosensation, and vestibular), processing that input, and scaling an appropriate motor response (i.e. muscle activation or strategy).

MOBILITY

The ability to navigate one's environment including obstacles. This includes tasks such as getting out of a chair; getting down onto and up off of the floor; gait tasks such as stepping up, over, and around obstacles or turning; accelerating and decelerating; and even running.

COGNITIVE/EMOTIONAL

A mix of cognitive tasks such as remembering information (memory), responding quickly to stimuli (processing speed), being able to focus on an object, task, or thought (attention), and performing more complex mental operations (executive function). This domain also includes the emotional aspects, such as a person's confidence in performing a task (self-efficacy) and mood state.

Each of these domains is, to a certain degree, distinct and separate from the others. However, there is a dynamic integration between them with some domains being more connected to others. For example, consider the Mobility Domain, which encompasses a person's ability to navigate their environment such as getting up and down from the floor, stepping over obstacles, turning quickly, etc. In some ways, an individual's mobility capabilities are dependent on all of the other domains. If a person lacks strength they may not be able to get out of a chair, much less off of the floor. If they lack cardiovascular endurance, then they may fatigue quickly, which may prevent them from navigating safely. Balance is obviously very closely tied to mobility. Neuromuscular issues could definitely impair a person's mobility, as will cognitive problems.

You can think of this model much like you would a good old-fashioned, homemade, Southern cherry pie. Imagine that pie hot and steaming right out of the oven. Now cut it into six pieces to represent the six domains. On the surface there are obviously six distinct pieces that you can identify, just like the domains have very specific definitions and characteristics. However, under the crust of the pie is a different story. If you try to get one of those pieces onto your plate, you had better move that plate as close to the pie pan as you can because you are going to have to quickly whip that piece onto your plate. Otherwise, all of the filling is just going to ooze right out and all you will be left with is a couple pieces of crust. So, although there were six pieces on the surface, there was still just one big pie underneath. That is how these six domains operate. They are distinct on the surface but they are also dynamically interconnected below it.

The recognition of these factors (both the domains and sub-domains) is critical to maximizing function as we age. Understanding their relationship with one another and targeting them with specific exercises are what characterizes "functional training." In this approach to exercise, movement challenges are utilized that attempt to maximize a person's ability to perform real-life tasks with greater ease and, ideally, with less pain and discomfort. So, the end goal isn't aesthetics or weight loss or even better disease management (although all of these may very well happen) but rather a person's "doability"—how it impacts their ability to do all of the stuff they need and like to do. What a person needs or wants to be able to do can vary widely, as we discussed earlier. But what is preventing them from performing those tasks can also vary widely.

Consider again the Functional Trajectory of Aging. That image represents an individual's overall level of functioning. However, think about a trajectory for each of the six domains of function. What is your current level and future trajectory of muscle strength? What is your current level and future trajectory of cardiorespiratory endurance? What is your current level and future trajectory of balance? Etcetera. The trajectory of these domains varies widely between individuals so that even people of similar overall functional abilities may have different deficits in these factors. One individual may have lost a significant amount of strength (i.e. a strength deficit), while another individual may have adequate strength but has lost a significant amount of coordination. Of course, the practical implication is that they will not benefit equally from the same types of exercises. For the first person, spending time strength training could really help them do more but it wouldn't likely make much of a difference for the second person.

As the research suggests, the optimal exercise program for an individual is one that addresses their individual areas of weakness (i.e. their deficits). This is, in many ways, reflective of the Principle of Specificity discussed earlier. Certain tasks are dependent on specific factors and, if an individual lacks adequacy in those factors, they will be unable to perform the task well. This doesn't mean that a general non-specific exercise program won't be beneficial. On the contrary, it could still be very valuable—it just might not be optimal.

Exercise is powerful. Our bodies and minds thrive on physical movement. The numerous benefits of even the most basic exercise routine for older adults have been well documented. Even the exercise guidelines for older adults are pretty basic, stating that everyone should perform cardiovascular exercise for about 30 minutes most days of the week and complete a couple sessions of strength training weekly. Not too complicated. Frankly, I wish more people would at least follow this minimal approach to exercise because it would be very beneficial for a lot of people. Exercise is powerful, and there is a tremendous amount of research showing that just going from nothing to something is helpful. But I also know that it would not solve many people's issues nor reverse their current downward trajectory because, while beneficial, it is not an optimal approach since it does not target an individual's specific needs.

Consider an inactive person with balance issues who has become a little more unsteady on their feet over the past few years. A generic exercise program, such as the minimal approach described above, will definitely provide lots of great benefits, but it won't address their main issue since basic cardiovascular and strength training have very little to no impact on balance. In order for them to improve their balance they would need to consistently perform exercises that challenge their balance in lots of different ways. It would be even more effective if they were to perform an in-depth evaluation of their balance systems in order to find out what types of balance exercises would be most beneficial. The more targeted the program can be, the better the results will be.

FUNCTIONAL LEVELS

According to the Hierarchy of Functional Aging (credit: Functional Aging Institute), there are eight categories of functional abilities—Frail; Pre-Frail; Lower Independent; Higher Independent; Semi-Fit; Fully Fit; and Elite—and they represent a continuum from the least functional to the most functional. Therefore, even though there are eight distinct categories, individuals in the same category can still differ. For example, someone in the higher independent category may be at the top end of scores for that group while another person is at the bottom end of scores. So even within each category, there is variability that must be taken into consideration.

As you read through the descriptions of each category below, make an honest self-assessment of which level best reflects your abilities and lifestyle. If you are having a tough time choosing between two levels, then choose the lower one just to be on the conservative side.

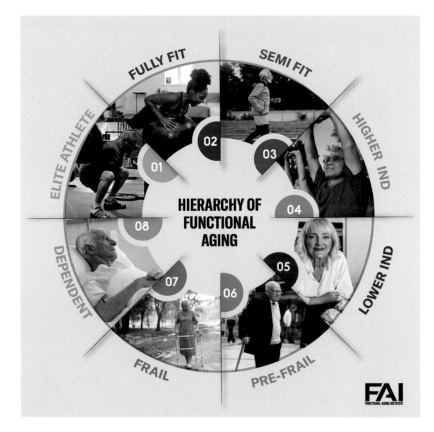

HIERARCHY OF FUNCTIONAL AGING

Elite: The physically elite have achieved and maintained the highest levels of physical function in their age group and are often more fit than sedentary or insufficiently active individuals that are decades younger. Compared to others their age and gender, the elite typically score in the top 1 to 5 percent of scores on functional and physical fitness tests. They train rather intensely on a regular basis and often compete in tournaments, races, and events. Due to their high levels of activity (and usually excellent dietary habits), they are also typically in excellent health, although this is not guaranteed and is somewhat dependent on how long they have been a regular exerciser. In the oldest age groups (85+ and 100+) in competitive sports, there are many individuals who did not start training until they were in their 60's or 70's, while others have been active and even competing since they were young.

Fully Fit: Fully fit older adults exercise primarily for their health and well-being rather than for competition and do so on a regular basis. Their exercise program is typically less intense and of shorter duration than the physically elite, and while they may still include sport-specific training in their routine, it is typically more for enjoyment than for true competition. The fully fit also enjoy higher than average levels of health and are typically estimated to be much younger than their chronological age by their peers. Fully fit individuals exceed the capabilities of others their own age in almost every category of fitness, although they do not reach the performance levels of being considered elite. When considering age and gender matched performance norms, they will score in the top 5 to 10 percent across the board.

EXERCISE FOR THE ELITE AND FULLY FIT

The focus for these individuals will be ensuring that they are training properly and safely for longevity, including addressing factors outside of exercise. They can, and often do, engage in a wide variety of training modalities at a high level. It is important, therefore, that they are utilizing proper techniques and planning their training program intelligently to avoid injury and over-training. In addition, factors such as nutrition, hydration, sleep, and recovery methods should be addressed, as they can either support or hinder their performance.

Semi-Fit: This group of older adults differs from the fully fit individuals by only having one or two areas of fitness in which they excel rather than excelling in most or all of the areas. This is usually due to the fact that they exercise using only one modality. For example, swimmers or joggers may have really high levels of cardiorespiratory fitness, but their levels of muscle strength and balance may be at critically low levels. They are also typically of good to excellent health. When considering age and gender-matched performance norms, they will typically score in the top 5 to 10 percent in 1 or 2 categories of fitness.

EXERCISE FOR THE SEMI-FIT

Adding variety to the training program is the priority here, as these folks are already exercising consistently using at least one modality. Use the 6 Functional Domains as a template for training. This often means the person will need to cut down on their preferred mode of training in order to make time for other modes of training—a task that is sometimes difficult to accomplish. Don't let your high level of fitness in one domain deceive you into thinking you excel in all domains.

Higher Independent: These individuals can range from being typically physically active but not exercise on a regular basis to exercising on a regular basis but being rather inactive otherwise to being active and exercising regularly. If they do exercise it is typically a basic program (e.g. walking and a circuit of strength training machines), of lower intensity, and of limited variability. Leisure-time activities may include walking, hiking, yard work, gardening, tennis, golf, and the like. Their health may range from good to excellent typically without any serious debilitating disease (although they may have chronic diseases that they are managing and their disease may cause a rapid decline in function if it progresses) and, for the most part, they are fully functional. However, since they are not "fit," their physiological and functional reserves are more limited than those in the categories above. In general, individuals in this category are much more diverse compared to their more fit counterparts, with scores ranging from average to somewhat above average on typical measures of fitness. Their specific areas of "deficit" (see the 6 Domains of Function) also vary considerably.

Lower Independent: These individuals are typically minimally active or completely sedentary, often choosing hobbies and activities that require very little physical demand, such as reading. Due to their relative inactivity, they score below average on most functional fitness assessments and are at a higher risk of functional decline. This results in a steeper downward functional trajectory compared to higher independent or fit individuals. The lack of movement puts them at increased risk of developing serious chronic conditions and becoming frail or disabled.

EXERCISE FOR THE INDEPENDENT CLIENT

Heterogeneity is the word for this group as their strengths and deficits vary widely, even among people with seemingly similar functional abilities. For one individual, their deficit may be strength and power while another individual may be sufficient in these areas but low in balance and mobility. It is important for them to try different types of movements to help identify areas in which they struggle. If they never perform an agility exercise, for example, then they may never discover that they struggle with those types of movements.

Pre-Frail: This is a critical transitional stage between independence and frailty that is characterized by meeting 1 or 2 of the 5 frailty criteria listed in the section on frail individuals below (frail individuals must meet 3 or more). These individuals score lower than average on all functional fitness assessments and are on a steep downward functional trajectory toward frailty and dependence if the appropriate interventions are not made. Due to their low physical ability levels, it is difficult for them to engage in instrumental activities of daily living (IADL's) such as shopping, yard work, house work, and leisure activities. Therefore, they continue to become less active and less engaged in life (occupational, social, recreational). This can quickly become a downward spiral: less activity leads to reduced physical abilities, which leads to less physical activity, and so on and so forth.

Frail: According to Campbell and Buchner (1997), frailty is a "condition or syndrome that results from a multi-system reduction in reserve capacity to the extent that a number of physiological systems are close to, or past, the threshold of symptomatic clinical failure. As a consequence, the frail person is at increased risk of disability and death from minor external stresses." The criteria for diagnosing frailty include three or more of the following characteristics:

1. Unintended weight loss (at least 10 lbs or >5% body weight in prior year);
2. Muscle weakness (grip strength in lowest 20 percent for gender and BMI);
3. Exhaustion or poor endurance;
4. Slow gait speed (typically a usual gait speed of less than 0.8m/s); and
5. Low levels of physical activity.

Sarcopenia (significant loss of muscle mass and strength due to aging) is a central feature of frailty and is of critical importance. Frail older adults can perform most or all basic activities of daily living (BADL's) such as bathing, dressing, transferring, toileting, and feeding, although they are typically unable to perform all of the instrumental activities of daily living (IADL's) such as shopping, doing laundry, preparing meals, and doing light housework. Since many frail older adults have difficulty ambulating, the use of assistive devices (canes, walkers, and rollers) is common. Frail older adults are at high risk of suffering from an injurious fall; are more likely to have osteoporosis; and typically qualify for physical therapy services due to their condition.

EXERCISE FOR THE FRAIL AND PRE-FRAIL CLIENT

Developing strength and power is the priority, since sarcopenia is the central feature of the frailty syndrome. While this group will have balance, mobility, and gait deficits, it is recommended to work on strength/power first to enable balance, mobility, and gait training. Simple machine-based and/or isolated movements are recommended at first before moving to more whole-body functional moves. For example, work on leg press, leg curl, and leg extension in order to facilitate a chair stand, which can then lead to a squat pattern. There will be a transitional time when they may be alternating between these movements from session to session. Shoot for a moderate to high intensity load for 8 to 12 repetitions. Another important component is regular physical activity, such as walking, outside of training. These folks should shoot for 30 to 60 minutes of moderate intensity movement every day.

Dependent: These individuals are unable to perform all of the BADL's and are dependent on others and/or physical aids (e.g. canes, walkers, wheelchairs) to complete their daily tasks. The extent of their physical disability is determined by the degree to which they cannot perform BADL's and IADL's. Disability rates increase with chronological age and are higher in females, African Americans, and the poor. Individuals can move in and out of disablement such as following a stroke (where function is lost) and during rehabilitation (where function is often regained). It is unlikely that fitness professionals will train dependent older adults unless they work in a nursing home or assisted living facility.

So, where do you stack up on the hierarchy? What level do you feel describes you the best? If you feel undecided between two levels then choose the lower level, as it is always better to start conservatively.

What do you want to do?

Having a better understanding of where you currently stand functionally is a great starting point for putting together a program that is going to give you optimal results. The other part of the equation is determining what it is that you want to be able to do. Are you okay with just being able to live independently and putter around the yard without fearing you might fall and hurt yourself? Or do you want to be able to downhill ski until you are 100? The exercise program required to downhill ski is going to look a *lot* different, because skiing is a lot more difficult than basic yard work.

John, now in his late 60's, had recently completed physical therapy following double knee replacements. He came into the fitness facility somewhat despondent because his surgeon had told him he would need to give up snow skiing. This hit him pretty hard because it was his favorite activity. Well, it was actually much more than that. John had grown up skiing and it was now one of his family's greatest activities to do together. He owned two ski-out chalets, each at a different ski resort. He, his wife, his adult kids, and his grandkids would spend a week at each resort every winter. Plus, he and his wife, or sometimes he and his buddies, would regularly hit the slopes over a weekend. These ski trips had made for some incredible memories and, only being in his 60's, he wanted to see that tradition continue for as long as possible. Give up skiing? Unthinkable! What would you do?

John was determined to get back to skiing despite his doctor's recommendations. He had the rest of his life to live. The knee replacements had been successful at removing his joint pain and so now it was just a matter of getting back into shape. As you can imagine, training to downhill ski again required a more robust and intense training program than is typical. At first, his program focused on basic strength and power, flexibility, and balance. By the end there was a lot of jumping, bounding, lateral movements, dynamic balance exercises, and more weight lifting involved. Before his knee replacement, John was definitely on the lower end of the fully fit category so his recovery went well with no issues and he took to training like a fish to water. I am happy to say that John was able to get back to the slopes (although gently at first) and continued to make more memories with his family and friends.

Does everyone need to train as robustly and intensely as John? Only if everyone wants to be able to ski black diamonds. If not, then you need to figure out what it is you are wanting to accomplish. This way you can map out where you are now compared to where you want to be in a year or 5 years or 10 or 20. And don't sell yourself short on your dreams. You may surprise yourself on how capable you become after just a few short months.

So now that you have a much better handle on what functional training is all about, including the Six Domains of Function and the Hierarchy of Functional Aging, we can focus on exercise strategies and movements. In the following chapters we will specifically focus on Cardiovascular Exercise; Strength and Power Movements; and Balance and Mobility exercises. Each of these is an important area to include in your exercise program. Each chapter will address some of the evidence regarding benefits, tackle essential concepts, and address specific movements. Later, I will explain more about how to put a program together using these exercises that hones in on your specific needs so that you get the most out of your exercise program.

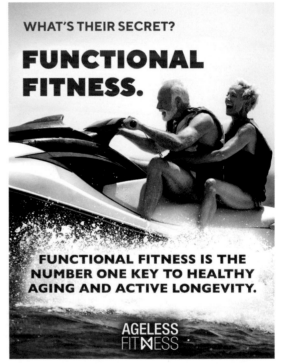

CHAPTER 3
Exercises for Cardiovascular Endurance

In some societies, like in the Blue Zones, physical activities are built right into the fabric of society, so there is almost no need to actually exercise formally. In these special places people have to walk, bike, hike, climb, and carry on a daily basis, which doesn't stop as they get older. Unfortunately, in most modern societies people typically engage in less physical activity overall, which gets worse the older they become. These societies are really built on reducing our need for movement in general. I remember the days when we had to (gasp!) walk to the TV to change the channel! Oh, the horrors! Thank goodness I can now sit on my duff for hours on end bingeing one episode after another without ever moving from my spot, thanks to my trusty friend the remote control.

Because we just don't move enough, naturally there is a dire need for formal exercise as we get older, which includes aerobic (cardiovascular) exercise. Aerobic exercise has been shown to be one of the most effective activities for decreasing risk of almost all chronic diseases; managing many current diseases better; and increasing cardiovascular fitness (Chodzko-Zajko et al 2009). It can reduce blood pressure, mitigate stress, improve insulin sensitivity, prevent weight gain, aid weight loss, and keep our brains healthy. Did you know that aerobic exercise is just as effective as some medications for mild depression? Plus, it has long been associated with longevity.

Here are the basic cardiovascular exercise recommendations for older adults:

Frequency: Most, preferably all, days of the week
Intensity: 60 to 90 percent max heart rate
             OR 12 to 15 RPE (Rating of Perceived Exertion)

Time:	30+ min
Type:	Your choice

Ultimately, the goal is to accumulate 150+ minutes of moderate-intensity cardiovascular exercise each week OR 75+ minutes of high-intensity exercise OR a combination of the two (each high-intensity minute is worth 2 moderate-intensity minutes). Let's break this down a little further.

INTENSITY: HOW HARD?

Cardiovascular exercise should be of sufficient intensity (> 60 percent max heart rate) in order to improve cardiovascular fitness and achieve optimal health benefits. This does not mean that exercising at a lower intensity isn't beneficial. As a matter of fact, anyone who is really deconditioned should probably start at an even lower intensity. Maximal heart rate is typically calculated as 220 – age but more recent information indicates that a more accurate equation for determining maximal heart rate is 208 – (0.7 x age) in healthy adults over the age of 40 (Tanaka et al 2001). The original formula tends to overestimate maximal heart rate in younger populations and underestimate them for older populations. Then, simply multiply that number by the intensity (i.e. 60 percent) to find out where your exercising heart rate should be. You can use a smart watch to measure your heart rate or take it yourself by finding the pulse in your neck (just beside your Adam's apple) using two fingers laid flat. Count the number of pulses over a period of 30 seconds and multiply by two to get beats per minute.

PREDICTED HEART RATE BY AGE AND INTENSITY

	50	55	60	65	70	75	80	85	90
100%	172	169	165	162	158	155	151	148	145
90%	155	152	149	146	142	140	136	133	131
80%	138	135	132	130	126	124	121	118	116
70%	120	118	116	113	111	109	106	104	102
60%	103	101	99	97	95	93	91	89	87
50%	86	85	83	81	79	78	76	74	73

Other methods, such as the "talk test" or rating of perceived exertion (RPE) are also valuable and actually much easier for most people to use. If you are taking medications that suppress heart rate such as beta blockers, then other methods are preferable. The Talk Test is very simple. If you can hold a conversation without having to pause often to catch your breath, then the exercise is too easy. If you can barely hold a conversation because you are so out of breath, then the exercise is too difficult. Find the balance where you can still speak some but not continuously.

The Rating of Perceived Exertion (RPE) scale is a 6- to 20-point scale that ranges from very easy (6) to maximal effort (20). An RPE of 12 to 13 represents moderate intensity exercise, while 15 to 17 represents high-intensity exercise. RPE is often an easier tool to use when heart rate monitors are unavailable and counting a pulse rate is difficult. You simply look at the scale and point at the number that corresponds to how difficult you feel the exercise is for you. Surprisingly, RPE ratings correspond very closely to heart rate, so this is an easy alternative to measuring heart rate.

BORG RATINGS OF PERCEIVED EXERTION (RPE) SCALE

RATINGS	PERCEIVED EXERTION
6	
7	Very Very Light
8	
9	Very Light
10	
11	Fairly Light
12	
13	Somewhat Hard
14	
15	Hard
16	
17	Very Hard
18	
19	Very Very Hard
20	

Source: https://borgperception.se/obtain-a-license-for-research-and-education/

HOW LONG AND HOW OFTEN?

Frequency and duration (time) are also important variables to consider so that you can reach the recommended volume of exercise each week. The good news is that you don't actually have to complete 30 minutes of exercise at one time. Studies show that three bouts of 10 minutes are just as beneficial as 30 minutes all at once. For many people, shorter bouts fit into their schedules a lot easier. The key is that the exercise must be of sufficient intensity. Cramped for time? Take a brisk walk before breakfast, a quick hike around noon, and a bike ride after dinner.

WHAT SHOULD I DO?

How do you like to move—walk, hike, swim, bike, row? Almost anything is an option as long as it is sustained activity that sufficiently elevates your heart rate. Try new activities until you find some options that you enjoy. Some people love to walk on a treadmill while others want to be outside. But you won't know until you try both. There are very likely some options that you haven't tried before. Don't let the fear of the unknown stop you. Find someone who knows how to do it and have them show you. Then give it a go a few times. However, your choice should also be driven by what is most appropriate for your physical conditions and, more specifically, your orthopedic conditions. Individuals without significant health risks or orthopedic conditions can typically participate in more high-impact exercises such as basketball or running. Those with orthopedic concerns, such as significant arthritis of the knees, hips, or spine; joint replacements; osteoporosis, etc. should avoid high-impact exercises and instead opt for low- or non-impact exercises such as bicycling, swimming, stationary bike, recumbent bike, recumbent stepper, treadmill, elliptical trainer, and rower. Clients with a history of falling or with balance deficits should avoid activities that have an increased risk of falling such as skiing or skating.

START WHERE YOU ARE

If you have not been performing aerobic exercise regularly then start on the low end of intensity and focus on getting the recommended volume (150+ minutes) first. Then you can gradually increase intensity into the moderate and moderate-high zones. When it comes to improving cardiovascular fitness, intensity is king, but any sustained movement is beneficial even at lower intensity levels. So, although moderate-intensity exercise is generally recommended for most people, your health conditions, fitness status, and goals will determine the appropriate level of intensity that is both safe and effective for you. If you are already accustomed to aerobic exercise, then one method you should consider using is High-Intensity Interval Training (HIIT).

KICK IT UP A NOTCH WITH HIGH-INTENSITY INTERVAL TRAINING (HITT)

This form of training simply involves intervals of higher-intensity exercise alternated with periods of lower-intensity exercise (recovery periods) within the same exercise session. How challenging and how long these periods last vary depending on the person's goals and abilities. Typically, they are prescribed as a ratio such as 3:1 (e.g. 3 minutes of higher-intensity followed by 1 minute of low-intensity recovery) or 2:1 (e.g. 60 seconds of higher-intensity followed by 30 seconds of recovery) or even 1:12 (e.g. 10 seconds of all-out effort followed by 120 seconds of rest). The more intense the exercise, the shorter it needs to be (because intense exercise cannot be sustained for very long) and the longer the rest period (in comparison to the exercise interval period) needs to be. Think about it this way. An all-out sprint of 100 yards would take the average individual about 15 to 20 seconds. But they would get so out of breath that they would need to rest for about 2 to 3 minutes or longer before they would be ready for the next sprint. That would be a ratio of 1:8 to 1:12. Conversely, if you just jogged the same distance and took 30 to 45 seconds to do so you might only need a minute before you were ready to jog again because you wouldn't get out of breath nearly as much. That would be a ratio of only 1:2.

How does it work? During the exercise intervals (periods of high-intensity exercise), heart rate and metabolism increase significantly. During the periods of recovery (lower-intensity exercise), heart rate, oxygen usage, and metabolism remain elevated above the level that you would expect from the low-intensity exercise. Imagine if you had to run (or walk briskly) a couple blocks in order to catch up to a friend. Once you got there you would be breathing hard with your heart pounding fast in your chest and it would take several minutes of rest before they recovered to normal levels. Even though you are standing still, you are burning way more calories compared to what you were burning while standing still before the little run. We call this extra calorie usage "the afterburn."

THE AFTERBURN

Here is a principle you need to remember: The greater the intensity during the workout, the greater the afterburn. It is kind of like shaking a snow globe. If you give it just a little shake then you don't disturb all of the flakes and the snow disappears quickly. But if you give it a vigorous shake, you disturb many more flakes and with the water swirling violently around inside it takes much longer for the snow to disappear. Exercise "shakes up" your metabolism and the harder you exercise the more calories you burn afterwards.

In addition, the afterburn specifically targets fat calories due to an interesting physiological mechanism called the crossover effect. As you are aware, during high-intensity aerobic exercise the body uses more calories, as a percentage, from carbohydrates than from fat in the body. During lower-intensity exercise, the body uses more calories, as a percentage, from fat than from carbohydrates in the body. It is easy to be misled in thinking then that lower-intensity exercise would be better for fat loss because more fat is used as energy. However, that is false for two reasons. The first reason is that although the body uses a lower percentage of calories from fat during higher-intensity exercise, it burns calories much faster so this partially offsets the change in percentage. Secondly, because of the afterburn, following high-intensity aerobic exercise that uses lots of carbohydrates, your body decides to save as much carbohydrate as it can and switches (or crosses over) to using fat as an energy source. Since the afterburn has been shown to last for 24 hours or more, then you end up burning a lot more fat *after* the exercise session than you did *during* the exercise session. The crossover effect combined with the afterburn is a very powerful 1-2 punch for losing body fat.

The advantages of HIIT training compared to traditional sustained cardiovascular exercise are that higher-intensity exercise leads to greater gains in cardiorespiratory fitness and it is time-efficient so workouts can be shorter. HIIT also seems to lead to greater loss of body fat and may provide some advantages for other aspects of metabolic health.

HIIT PROGRAM BASICS

Rating of Perceived Exertion (RPE) is a useful way to gauge intensity during HIIT rather than heart rate because it is much simpler and doesn't require any math or pulse counting. Ideally RPE should reach 16 to 19 during the higher-intensity intervals and 9 to 12 during the lower-intensity intervals. Intensity, duration, and recovery are interdependent. The harder the exercise interval, the shorter the client will be able to do it and the longer recovery period they will require. So, you may only be able to last

30 seconds at an RPE of 19 and require 3 minutes to recover but you may be able to last two minutes at an RPE of 17 and only require one minute to recover.

To increase intensity during the intervals you can go faster with light resistance (sprints), slower with high resistance (climbs), or faster with moderate resistance (hills). The combinations of challenges (sprints, climbs, and hills), intensities, interval periods, rest periods, and total workout time creates a virtually endless array of combinations, so you really never even have to perform the exact same routine twice to get amazing results.

HIIT FOR THE BEGINNER

Here are some tips for those that are new to HIIT or are out of shape:

- Choose the cardio exercise that you feel the most comfortable with (treadmill, outdoor walking, stationary bike, elliptical, seated stepper, etc.)
- Experiment by exercising a little harder than usual until you feel like you are getting out of breath and then back off to your usual pace or even a little below it
- Note how you feel during the recovery period, and when you have caught your breath then try it again
- Use longer intervals (2 to 3 minutes) and limit how hard you go during the higher-intensity intervals (RPE 16-17)
- The length of the recovery intervals should be longer than the higher-intensity intervals; shoot for a ratio of 1:2 or 1:3
- When you feel comfortable, try one of our sample beginner routines

BEGINNER HIIT WORKOUT # 1
Total time: 20min

Warm-Up (4:00) – Start easy and gradually increase exercise intensity so that you achieve an RPE of about 11-12 (this is your base level) by the end of the warm-up.

Stage 1 (9:00) 3 Hills
Hill #1: Increase speed and resistance/incline to an RPE of 15 for 1 minute. Return to base level for 2 minutes.
Repeat twice.

Stage 2 (4:00) 3 Sprints
Sprint #1: Increase speed only to an RPE of 17 for 20 seconds. Return to base level for 60 seconds.
Repeat twice.

Cool-Down (3:00) – Decrease intensity to achieve an RPE of 9-10. Heart rate should return to within about 20 to 30 beats per minute of pre-exercise value.

BEGINNER HIIT WORKOUT #2
Total time: 25min

Warm-Up (4:00) – Start easy and gradually increase exercise intensity so that you achieve an RPE of about 11-12 (this is your base level) by the end of the warm-up.

Stage 1 (12:00) 3 Climbs
Hill #1: Increase resistance/incline to an RPE of 15 for 2 minutes. Return to base level for 2 minutes.
Repeat twice.

Extra Recovery (1:00) – Stay at base level or adjust accordingly so that you are fully recovered for the next challenge.

Stage 2 (4:00) 4 Sprints
Sprint #1: Increase speed to an RPE of 17 for 20 seconds. Return to base level for 40 seconds.
Repeat three times.

Cool-Down (3:00) – Decrease intensity to achieve an RPE of 9-10. Heart rate should return to within about 20 to 30 beats per minute of pre-exercise value.

HIIT FOR THE EXPERIENCED
Here are some tips for those who already perform cardio exercise on a regular basis and are in good shape:

- Try out one of the sample beginner programs to see how you respond
- Choose any mode of exercise that you are accustomed to, but don't be afraid to experiment with new forms. For example, if you are having a difficult time challenging yourself while walking outside but don't want to jog or run (maybe due to joint issues), then try the elliptical trainer (allows greater increases in intensity while still being gentle on the joints)
- Play with the intervals and intensities to find out what works best for you and what you enjoy the most
- Mix up your HIIT routine so that you aren't always doing to same thing—keep it fresh and interesting; the possibilities are endless

ADVANCED HIIT WORKOUT
Total Time: 32:30 min

Warm-Up (4:00) – Start easy and gradually increase exercise intensity so that you achieve an RPE of about 11-12 (this is your base level) by the end of the warm-up.

Stage 1 (7:30)
Sprint for 2 min at RPE 18 with 30 sec recovery
Hill for 2 min at RPE 18 with 30 sec recovery
Sprint for 2 min at RPE 18 with 30 sec recovery

Extra Recovery (1:00)

Stage 2 (5:00)
Hill for 1 min at RPE 18 and 1 min at RPE 19-20 with 30 sec recovery
Repeat

Extra Recovery (1:00)

Stage 3 (11:00)
Hill for 3 min at RPE 17 with 60 sec recovery
Max sprint for 30 sec with 60 sec recovery
Repeat twice

Cool-Down (3:00) – Decrease intensity to achieve an RPE of 9-10. Heart rate should return to within about 20 to 30 beats per minute of pre-exercise value.

CARDIOMETABOLIC RESISTANCE TRAINING

Another effective and efficient method to increase the intensity of your workouts is to perform resistance and cardiovascular exercises in rapid succession in order to simultaneously improve strength and cardiovascular endurance—a style of training that has been widely popularized by CrossFit, but don't let that scare you. There are many different ways to do this and several are briefly described below.

- Every Minute On the Minute (EMOM) – Perform a set number of repetitions of a specific movement as quickly as you can. Rest until the minute is over and perform another exercise in the same fashion. If it takes you 30 seconds to complete a set then you will have 30 seconds to rest before your next exercise. However, if it takes you 50 seconds to complete a set, then you only have 10 seconds of rest until starting the next movement. Regardless, this provides a brief rest in between each exercise. Continue until you reach a predetermined time limit.
- AMRAP (As Many Repetitions as Possible) – Select several movements and perform as many repetitions of each movement as you can within a set period of time. For example, for 30 seconds each, perform air squats, step ups, modified pushups, band rows, and kettlebell deadlifts. Repeat this sequence 3 or 4 times without rest.
- AMRAP (As Many Rounds as Possible) – Perform a set number of repetitions of a series of exercises (called a round). For example, one round may consist of 20 kettlebell swings, 20 squat jumps, 10 pushups, and a 200m run/jog. Repeat that same series of exercises as many times as you can within a set period of time, which can range anywhere from 10 to 30 minutes.

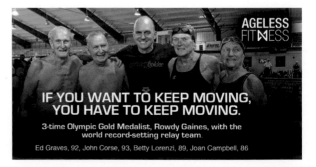

AGELESS FITNESS

IF YOU WANT TO KEEP MOVING, YOU HAVE TO KEEP MOVING.

3-time Olympic Gold Medalist, Rowdy Gaines, with the world record-setting relay team.

Ed Graves, 92, John Corse, 93, Betty Lorenzi, 89, Joan Campbell, 86

CHAPTER 4
Exercises for Strength and Power

Having inadequate levels of muscle mass and strength puts you at risk of future disability and even death, so if you aren't weight-lifting, then you need to start as soon as possible. It is probably the most important thing you can do to ensure you remain as physically capable as you can as you get older. Strength tends to decline rapidly with advancing age, typically accelerating after the age of 70, but the rate of decline is almost entirely dependent on your physical activity levels. For example, the typical sedentary 70-year-old may only have half the strength of a 40-year-old. However, the muscle of a 70-year-old triathlete is almost indistinguishable from that of a 40-year-old.

TEST YOUR STRENGTH

A quick and easy way to assess your lower body strength is the 30 Second Chair Stand Test. In this test, you will stand up from and sit down in a chair as many times as you can in 30 seconds. To perform this test, find a sturdy chair that is standard height (about 17 inches) that preferably does not have a padded seat. You will need a partner to time you.

Start by sitting upright in the middle of the chair with feet planted firmly on the floor shoulder-width apart. Cross your arms over your chest and keep them crossed the entire time. Have your partner give you the countdown or "Ready, Set, Go". On the word "go" stand up fully and then sit back down in the chair. Repeat this as many times as you can in 30 seconds. Be sure to actually sit down in the chair each time so that your weight shifts into the chair and to fully stand up each time as well.

Scoring

	60-69	70-79	80-89
Women	> 20 Excellent 18-19 Good 16-17 Okay 14-15 Weak <14 Very Weak	> 18 Excellent 16-17 Good 14-15 Okay 12-13 Weak < 12 Very Weak	> 17 Excellent 15-16 Good 13-14 Okay 11-12 Weak < 11 Very Weak
Men	> 22 Excellent 20-21 Good 18-19 Okay 16-17 Weak < 16 Very Weak	> 20 Excellent 18-19 Good 16-17 Okay 14-15 Weak < 14 Very Weak	> 17 Excellent 15-16 Good 13-14 Okay 11-12 Weak < 11 Very Weak

Reference: Adapted from the Senior Fitness Test Manual

Resistance training is often referred to as "weight lifting," but older adults can safely and effectively use a wide variety of equipment such as weight machines, resistance bands, free weights, body weight, hydraulic and pneumatic equipment. Equipment selection is dependent on the individual's capabilities and goals and what they have access to. Each type of equipment has its advantages and disadvantages, but even the most basic equipment can yield significant results. It is a misconception that older adults should only use light dumbbells or easy resistance bands because they might become injured. The muscles of older adults need to be challenged in order to grow just as the muscles of younger adults do and although this population has more orthopedic concerns than younger populations, resistance exercise has been shown to be generally safe.

This ageist stereotype that older adults should only lift light weights leads to an issue we refer to as "under dosing." This means that their muscles are not challenged enough to create a meaningful overload which significantly limits progress. Older adults *can* load heavy and there are benefits to doing so, but they don't *have to* load heavy because even more moderate loading schemes are also beneficial. It depends on the individual's abilities and goals.

STRENGTH AND POWER TRAINING MYTHS

1. Weight lifting is bad for your joints—actually, when done properly, getting stronger through lifting weights can reduce joint pain and inflammation during activities, enabling you to do more than you could previously.
2. Older adults shouldn't lift heavy weights—high and moderate loads have been found to be safe for older adults and effective for building strength.
3. Older adults shouldn't lift anything over their head—some people may have poor shoulder mobility and prior shoulder injuries that will make lifting weights overhead riskier. However, age should not be a limiting factor.
4. Strength training will make you "big and bulky"—this is true if you train hard and take steroids but otherwise it will just make you strong. Yes, you will increase your muscle mass, but not enough to be bulky.
5. Jumping is too risky—while it is definitely a riskier movement to perform for those with balance and significant joint issues, it is a valuable tool for improving strength, power, and function.
6. Moving fast and explosively will lead to injuries—you need to be able to move quickly, and the only way to get faster is to move faster. There is little evidence that performing fast, explosive movements increases injury rates.

It is clear that a strong relationship exists between muscle strength and functional abilities for older adults. In fact, it is widely considered the most important factor, which is why it is so important to build it. But how strong does a person need to be? Well, that depends. The relationship between strength and function starts to break down as a person's function improves. This means that individuals with the lowest levels of strength will benefit the most functionally from getting stronger. However, a person who has adequate levels of strength will not get that much benefit functionally from getting stronger. This phenomenon is called the "strength threshold."

Consider a person who barely has enough strength to get out of their chair. Getting stronger will likely have a significant effect on their ability to get out of a chair and it will become easier and easier to do so. At some point, however, the functional benefits from getting stronger will diminish. An individual who can squat 100 pounds can get out of a chair just as easily as someone who can squat 400 pounds. The second person is obviously a lot stronger, but this doesn't necessarily translate to improved functional ability unless, of course, you consider harder tasks that require more strength. Obviously, the stronger person will be able to lift heavier items with greater ease. For example, lifting a 40-pound bag of mulch or moving a wheelbarrow that is loaded down.

A LITTLE IS GOOD, BUT MORE IS BETTER

So, given this strength threshold effect, how strong does an older adult need to be? The answer: "Strong enough." Strong enough to perform the functional activities that are important to them. Since basic functional activities only require a minimal level of strength, some experts are advocating for a "minimal dose approach" for older adults in order to protect them from functional decline as they get older (Fisher et al 2017). This approach recommends a resistance training program with the following characteristics:

- Low frequency (2 days/week)
- Low time commitment (<30 min/session)
- Single set routine
- Simple machine-based exercises
- Low intensity (fatigue at 8-12 repetitions)

Many research studies have demonstrated improvements in muscle mass, strength, physical function, and a number of health variables by following this basic type of program. Muscle strength will likely improve slower than a more aggressive (higher loads, higher volume) program, but systematic reviews suggest that the most important long-term variables for improving muscle strength in older adults are exercise volume and duration of training (Raymond et al 2013; Borde, Hortobagyi and Granacher 2015). It is important to note this approach is recommended for adults who are still independent and therefore do not have major deficits in their muscle strength yet so the focus is on maintenance or slight improvement.

IT'S NEVER TOO LATE TO BUILD MUSCLE

An individual who has already lost a significant amount of muscle strength would likely need a more aggressive program than the "minimal dose approach" described above. Frail, pre-frail, and lower independent older adults often have significant strength deficits that are affecting their functional abilities. Improving their strength becomes a top priority, and any improvements will likely lead to improvements in function. Therefore, they may benefit more from a heavy loading scheme which research has shown time and time again is safe and effective for even the oldest and frailest. They may also benefit more from isolated strengthening due to deficits in balance, mobility, core/trunk stability, cognition, or other factors.

Following traditional progressive resistance training, the muscular strength of older adults can increase anywhere from 25 percent to more than 100 percent depending on the exercise program being used, the duration of the training, age and gender of the client, and the specific muscle groups being trained (Chodzko-Zajko et al 2009). It is generally recommended that mature adults engage in at least 2 days per week of moderate intensity strength training that includes 8 to 10 exercises involving the major muscle groups for 1 to 3 sets of 8 to 12 repetitions each (Chodzko-Zajko et al 2009).

The recovery period is an important aspect to consider. Some research has suggested that older adults need more than the typical 48-hour rest period in between resistance training sessions for any given muscle group. This means that training 2 days per week may be more effective than training 3 days per week for some individuals. An individual who is loading heavy is more likely to need a longer recovery period than the person using light or moderate loads. Varying the loads from session to session may also be beneficial for enhancing recovery.

Regardless of functional level, loaded multi-joint exercises may be the most beneficial for older adults as opposed to isolated exercises. Following a structured approach to multi-joint exercises, such as the 7 fundamental movement patterns described below, is an effective strategy.

7 FUNDAMENTAL MOVEMENT PATTERNS

1. Squat/Sit-to-stand
2. Hinge/Deadlift
3. Lunge/Step Up

4. Push/Press
5. Pull/Row
6. Anti-Rotation
7. Carry

These are all multi-joint patterns that can be performed in a variety of ways with different types of loads and are easily scaled to an individual's level of ability or modified according to specific chronic conditions.

DON'T LET AGE BE A BARRIER

It is a myth that a person should not (fill in the blank with an exercise) because of their age. You should not feel restricted from performing a movement pattern merely because you have reached some arbitrary age threshold. Restrictions should be based on your functional abilities, chronic conditions, and whether or not you have "earned the right" to perform that pattern. Earning the right means that you have the prerequisite mobility, stability, and movement pattern efficiency to load a pattern. For example, squatting is a great exercise that strengthens the lower body and trunk musculature and is a functional activity that is performed every day. Many people, young and old, have difficulty performing the squat correctly due to limitations in foot stability, ankle mobility, knee mobility, hip mobility, core stability, leg strength, hip strength, and/or thoracic mobility. And even if a person is sufficient in all of these areas, they still need to learn the squat pattern. These are the factors that determine whether or not someone has "earned the right" to load the squat…not their age.

You could argue that you will never have the necessary mobility and stability in all of these areas because your restrictions are too significant due to a lifetime of inactivity, past injuries or surgeries, the effects of chronic conditions (e.g. osteoarthritis, osteoporosis), or a combination of several of these. Therefore, you will never be able to perform a loaded squat pattern. This is not true. Every time you stand up from a chair then you are basically performing a loaded squat pattern using your body weight. There are many variations of these patterns that account for restrictions and will allow you to perform the movement to the best of your ability.

For example, if you have limited ankle mobility you will find it much easier to squat if you elevate your heels slightly or adopt a much wider, toe-out position. If you continue to fall backwards or lean too far forward during a squat you could perform a goblet squat (front-loaded squat using a kettle bell or dumbbell). If your knees collapse in during a squat, place a mini-band (resistance band loop) around your knees when squatting. And if you struggle with several restrictions, then simply loading the sit-to-stand is an appropriate alternative. There are many ways to perform these fundamental movement patterns no matter your age or ability level.

POWERFUL AGING

The term power training may bring to mind images of huge weight lifters in the Olympics wearing spandex overalls lifting hundreds of pounds over their heads, but this is not the type of power training covered here. Muscle power is a combination of strength and speed. In other words, as long as you are moving a weight (even just your body weight) fast, then you are working on power. So while traditional strength training, described earlier, utilizes slow and controlled movements, power training utilizes fast, explosive movements.

Many experts now believe that it is more important to develop power for older adults than it is to develop strength for a number of reasons. For one, muscle power declines earlier and faster than muscle strength with advancing age (Chodzko-Zajko et al 2009; Porter, 2006); power tends to be more important than muscle strength for performing many functional tasks such as stair-climbing and rising from a chair; and power training tends to be more effective at improving many functional abilities. These factors seem to apply across all levels of the functional hierarchy with possibly more significance for those on the lower end of function. Take tripping as an example. When a person trips while walking, a quick, powerful step is required in response in order to avoid falling. Without being fast enough to place a foot out in front of the body, then they will likely end up on the floor. Then, once their foot hits the ground, they will need to quickly create enough force to stop their body's movement. In this situation, being strong doesn't matter if there is insufficient speed and power.

You may believe, as many do, that moving fast would be dangerous. Dozens and dozens of studies with thousands of older adults confirm that power training is as safe as traditional strength training. Minor musculoskeletal discomfort (soreness) is the most commonly reported adverse event in the literature, although joint pain and falls are also potential concerns (Porter 2006). However, studies report no difference in adverse events between power training and strength training, with most injuries occurring during maximal power and strength testing. Power training has been used safely and effectively with a wide variety of older adults including the oldest-old, the frail, those with musculoskeletal conditions such as osteoarthritis and osteoporosis, and those with other disease conditions like Parkinson's disease, dementia, and post-stroke.

There are actually numerous additional benefits to power training over traditional strength training. Power training typically uses lighter loads so that the movement can be performed faster. The amount of weight and the speed of a movement are inversely related, meaning the greater the load, the slower you will be able to move it and the lighter the load the faster you will be able to move it. Lighter loads typically means less joint stress. It also means less muscle damage so recovery is faster. Plus, performing fast movements with lighter weight actually feels easier to do.

SO HOW DO YOU DO IT?

For power training to be truly effective, you need to perform a movement as fast as you can while keeping the best form possible. This is typically best accomplished by having a slow "loading" phase and then a fast "explosive" phase. For example, to perform Power Stands, you would sit in a chair and stand up as quickly as you can (explosive phase). Then you would sit back down slowly in a controlled manner (loading phase). Once seated, perform another stand as quickly as possible. This allows a person to focus on the explosive part while keeping good form. As with strength training, a wide variety of equipment including body weight, weighted vests, sand bags, medicine balls, resistance bands, free weights, aquatics, and pneumatic resistance exercise equipment can be used safely and effectively.

GUIDELINES FOR POWER TRAINING WITH MATURE ADULTS

1. Almost any of the 7 Fundamental Movement Patterns can be used for either strength or power training.
2. Perform 3 to 5 repetitions per set in order to maintain a greater velocity of movement and power output (de Vreede 2005) because power output drops off considerably after about the fourth or fifth repetition.
3. Prior to performing a movement explosively, learn and practice the proper technique using slow, controlled speeds, gradually speeding up the

movement to ensure you can maintain proper technique. If you cannot perform a movement accurately, then do not try to do it explosively.

4. Perform an appropriate warm-up before training by performing a movement at a moderate speed before trying to move as fast as possible.
5. Use lower loads (20 to 40 percent 1RM) and higher movement speeds.
6. Jumping (i.e. plyometric) exercises, such as squat jumps, are great for developing power, but there is a greater risk of falling and joint injuries during these movements. However, these types of explosive movements have been found to be both safe and effective for older adults (Moran et al. 2018). Practice proper jumping technique, including how to land softly, to ensure safety.
7. The primary focus of power training should be on lower-body musculature and tasks related to mobility, but upper-body muscle power may also be important for the maintenance of function (de Vreede et al 2005). Some movements naturally engage both lower and upper body musculature for generating power but the majority of power training exercises should involve the lower body.

POWER TRAINING EXERCISES

Just like with traditional strength training, power training movements can easily be scaled to your ability level so you can perform them safely. Power movements typically fall into four categories: Lifts; Throws; Jumps; and Start/Stop.

Lifts include traditional strength training movements such as leg press, leg extensions, squats, deadlifts, presses, pulls, etc. These can be performed with a variety of equipment such as weight stack machines, resistance bands, ankle straps, and free weights.

Throws include any type of movement when any object is thrown. This includes wall balls, slams, and chest passes, which are typically performed with some type of medicine ball. Since focusing on lower body power is more important, any type of throw should use the lower body to initiate and provide power to the throw.

Jumps include any movement where both feet leave the floor and are also known as plyometric exercises. They include hops, vertical jumps, broad/horizontal jumps, box jumps, skipping, bounding, etc. These are more appropriate for higher functioning individuals since they require adequate power and balance to be able to perform.

Studies have confirmed the safety and effectiveness of plyometric exercises for older adults. They suggest performing several different jumps 3 to 10 times for two to three sets each with about 60 seconds of recovery between sets. Do this for up to three training sessions per week in order to ensure effectiveness.

Balance becomes more difficult and risk of falling increases during some of the more dynamic power movements such as jumping. Learning how to jump and land safely and effectively may take some time, but you will get better as you practice.

<u>Starts and Stops</u> are walking/running exercises that require a person to accelerate and decelerate quickly. An example is the Red Light/Green Light game you may have played as a child. These types of exercises are performed without any external loading or equipment other than maybe a chair. The goal is for the client to either move as quickly as possible from a resting position or to stop as quickly as possible from a moving position.

Focusing on strength, speed, and power should be considered an essential part of a resistance exercise program for all levels of function. These can be easily performed at a gym, at home, or on the go.

STRENGTH AND POWER EXERCISES

BODYWEIGHT SQUAT

1. Stand with feet shoulder-width apart, or just a little wider, with toes pointed out slightly

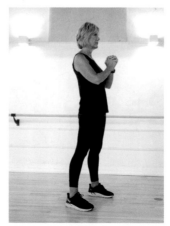

2. Bend at the hips, knees and ankles simultaneously to drop your bottom straight down towards your heels

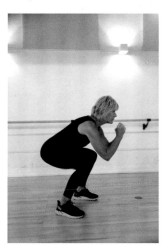

3. Drive your knees forward and slightly outward towards your little toe while keeping your heels on the ground as you squat down
4. Drop your bottom as low as possible, without pain, with the goal of getting your thighs to parallel with the floor or slightly lower
5. Your upper body will lean forward slightly but try to keep your chest facing forward as much as possible
6. Stand up by driving your feet into the ground and head towards the ceiling

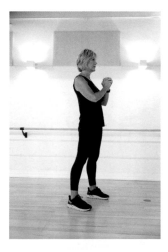

GOBLET SQUAT

1. Stand in the beginning squat position holding a dumbbell (DB) or kettlebell (KB) from the bottom with both hands keeping your elbows tucked in to your body and under the weight

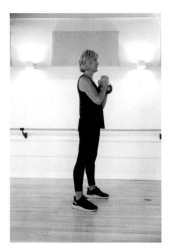

2. Follow the same steps to perform a squat with your elbows ending up inside your knees at the bottom

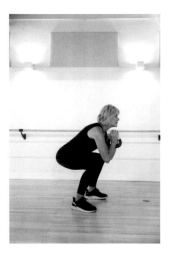

3. The weight will make it more challenging but may allow you to squat a little lower

Squat Tip: To develop more power, stand up as quickly as you can.

THRUSTER

1. Stand in the beginning squat position holding a DB in each hand by each shoulder

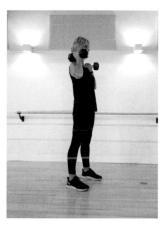

2. Perform the squat as described earlier

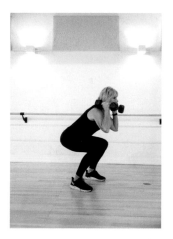

3. Stand up as quickly as you can using your lower body to drive the DB's over your head while straightening your arms

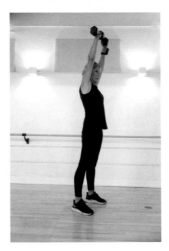

4. Lower the DB's back to shoulder height before squatting again

BOX/CHAIR SQUAT

1. Perform the same set up and movement as the squat but place a chair behind you so that the corner of the chair pokes between your legs

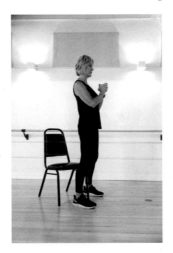

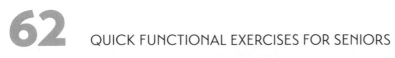

2. Squat down until your bottom touches the chair

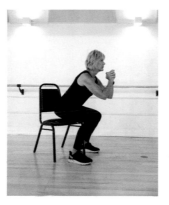

3. Do not sit down completely but keep some tension in your legs before standing back up

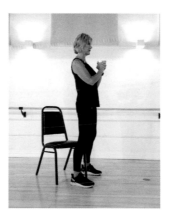

VERTICAL JUMP

This "squat" variation is great for developing power more so than the movements described earlier. While it may seem somewhat scary to try this at first it will become easier and easier as you get the hang of jumping and landing. To help ease you into jumping I have created a simple four step approach described below.

Step 1: Slowly go down into a squat position with arms reaching towards your heels or slightly behind them. Hold this position for 2-3 seconds while you try to get into good alignment (see instructions on Bodyweight Squat). Repeat this 8-10 times until you feel that your body can remember this position.

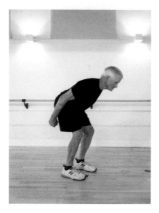

Step 2: Repeat as in Step 1 but go down into the squat position really quickly and hold the position. It may be difficult to go down quickly and end up in the correct squat position so always readjust yourself at the bottom. Hold that position for 2-3 seconds and then stand up. Keep trying to "hit" the correct squat position at the bottom when you go down quickly.

Step 3: Repeat as in Step 1 but after holding the bottom position for 3-4 seconds, stand up as fast as you can without coming up on your toes. As you stand up drive your hands up and over your head.

Step 4: Repeat as in Step 3 but do not hold the bottom position. Quickly go down and immediately stand back up as fast as you can while driving your arms overhead.

Step 5: Repeat as in Step 4 but this time jump off the ground by extending your feet. When you land immediately and quickly go down into a half-squat position (similar to Step 2). This will absorb the impact so you can land softly and will help you to maintain your balance.

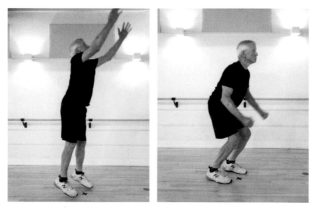

Once you get the hang of it, try to jump a little higher. Always take a second or two to reset in between jumps so that you can continue to use good form.

BAND SQUAT

1. Perform the same setup and movement as the squat
2. To add resistance, stand on a resistance tubing and hold the handles by your shoulders with the tubing running behind your arms
3. Keep your hands and elbows tucked in tight to your body during the entire movement

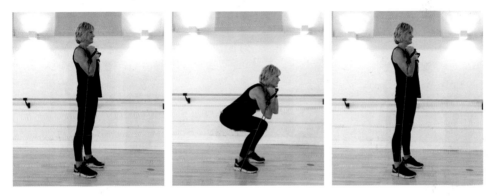

ROMANIAN DEADLIFT (AKA "RDL")

1. Stand with feet shoulder width apart holding a DB or KB in front of your body with both hands

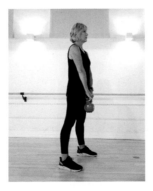

2. Keeping a slight bend in your knees, slide your hips back (as if you were shutting a file cabinet with your bottom)
3. Allow your trunk to fold forward so the weight drops straight down towards the middle of your feet until you feel that the back of your legs are "tight"

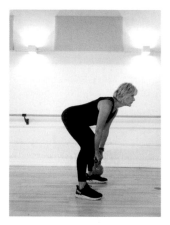

4. Do not bend your knees in order to go lower as you would in the traditional deadlift
5. While doing so contract your abdominal muscles so that your back does not round forward (squeezing your armpits with your arms will help)
6. Keep the weight close to your body so that it does not go past the end of your toes at any point
7. Drive your feet into the ground to stand back up (there is no need to take the weight all the way to the floor)

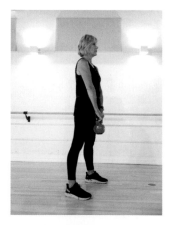

ROMANIAN DEADLIFT (AKA "RDL") WITH A SUPERBAND

1. Stand on a superband with your feet inside the loop
2. Reach down and grab the bottom of the loop and pull it taut

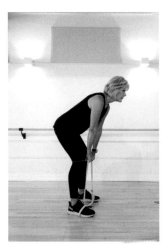

3. Establish a good starting deadlift position and perform the deadlift movement as described above

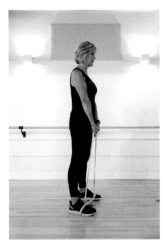

4. For added resistance, grab both the top and bottom of the loop

SINGLE LEG DEADLIFT

1. Stand with feet close together holding a DB or KB in one hand by your side
2. Bend forward at the waist to drop the weight towards the ground following the path of your stance leg while simultaneously reaching your opposite leg to the wall behind you
3. Keep a slight bend in your stance leg for balance
4. As with the previous deadlift patterns keep your trunk stiff so that it doesn't round forward
5. Stop when your torso and rear leg are parallel with the ground and then return to the standing position

Single Leg Deadlift Tip: This version requires a lot more balance so use the hand without the weight to lightly hold onto a stable object until you can do it without any assistance

WALKING LUNGE

1. Stand with feet shoulder width apart (optional: hold a DB in each hand by your sides)

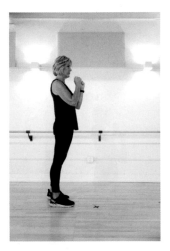

2. Step forward and bend your back knee until it touches the ground (touch it softly)

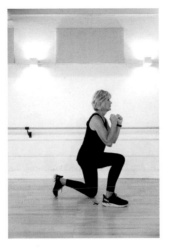

3. At this point your front and back legs should be at a 90-degree angle
4. Stand up by driving your front foot into the ground and bringing your back leg to your front leg (you will have taken one step forward)

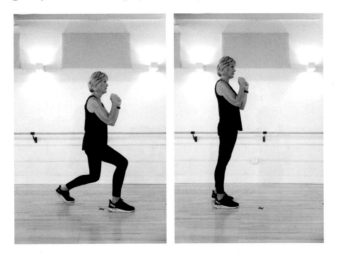

5. Try to keep your trunk in an upright position during the entire movement
6. Repeat by leading with the opposite leg

Lunge Tip: If doing a bodyweight lunge is too difficult you can use walking poles, the back of a couch, or chair seats to aid you.

STATIONARY LUNGE

1. Perform the same movement as the walking lunge except instead of stepping your back leg to your front leg you will stand up by pushing off of your front foot and returning it to your starting position (you will end up standing in the same spot)
2. Repeat with the other leg

Variation: Hold a weight in only one hand to provide an unbalanced load which will help to work on your core muscles and your balance.

GOBLET LUNGE

1. Stand with feet shoulder width apart holding a DB or KB from the bottom with both hands, keeping your elbows tucked in to your body and under the weight

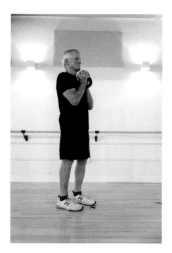

2. Perform either the walking or stationary lunge movement as described earlier

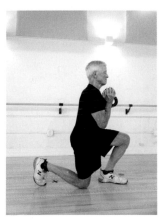

STEP-UPS

1. Stand in front of a step, sturdy box or bench with one leg on it

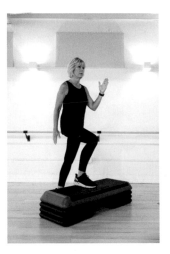

2. Your knee should be no higher than your hip, but start with a lower height if necessary

3. Step up onto the object with your back leg by focusing on driving your front leg down into the object

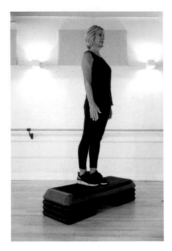

4. Try not to push off the back leg very much
5. As an option for more of a balance challenge, drive your back knee up into a marching position instead of placing it on the step

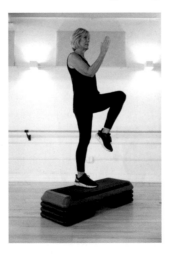

6. Repeat with the opposite leg

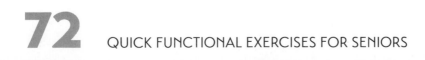

Variations: Hold DB's in one hand; Hold DB's in both hands; Hold DB or KB in the goblet position

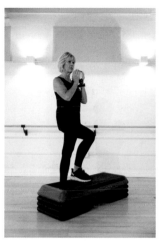

SIDE LUNGE

1. Begin in a standing position

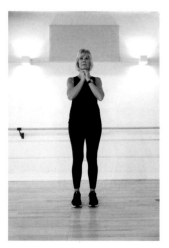

2. Take a large step sideways

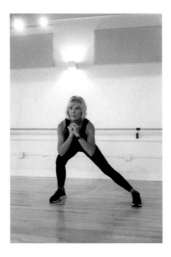

3. As your foot hits the ground, lower your bottom towards the heel of the stepping foot so that your weight shifts onto that leg
4. Your trail leg should straighten but stay on the floor for balance
5. Drop as low as you are able and then powerfully push off so that you can return to a standing position in one movement

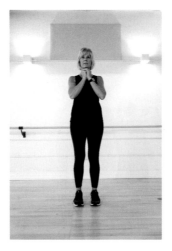

6. Repeat with the opposite leg

BUG STOMPS

This lunge variation will help to develop more speed and power which is useful for fall prevention as well as every day and sports performance.

1. From a standing position, imagine that there are huge bugs on the ground all around you

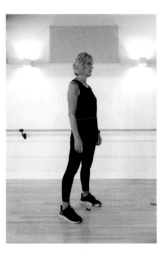

2. Stomp on the ground in front of you in a quick and powerful manner as if you were trying to squash a large bug

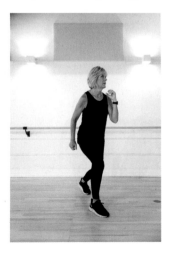

3. Most of your body weight should shift quickly onto the stomping leg
4. Return to the starting position and repeat with the other leg
5. Don't just stomp in the same place each time but vary the direction and distance you need to stomp
6. Focus on moving quickly and stomping hard on the bugs

POWER STEP

This variation builds on the bug stomp and takes it to the next level. It is the essence of fall prevention as we will all stumble, trip, or slip at some point and need to react in order to keep ourselves upright and safe.

1. From a standing position allow your entire body to start "falling" forward from your toes without bending at the waist

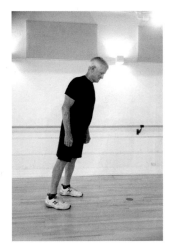

2. You will feel that there is a "point of no return" as your body falls forward so that if you don't react then you will fall flat on your face
3. Once you feel this happen quickly take a large and powerful step with your right foot (think a long bug stomp) and plant it firmly in the ground to stop your forward momentum

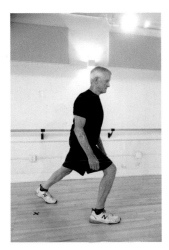

4. Return to the starting position and repeat by stepping forward with your left foot
5. This will be very uncomfortable at first so keep trying until you get it right
6. As always, be sure to be in a location where you could catch yourself if you do happen to fall

GLUTE BRIDGE

1. Lie on your back with knees bent and feet shoulder-width apart on the floor (you may use a small pillow or towel to support your head if necessary)

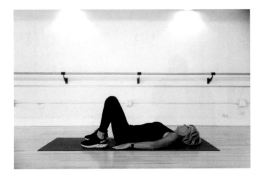

2. Place hands palms down by your sides

3. Drive your heels into the ground while pushing your hips to the ceiling until your body makes a straight line from your shoulders to your knees

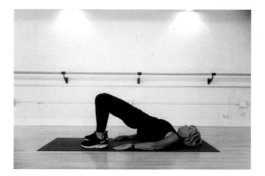

4. Hold this position for 5-10 seconds before lowering back down
5. Keep your head relaxed to avoid pushing the back of your head into the ground as this will strain your neck area

MARCHING GLUTE BRIDGE

1. Perform the same setup and movement as the glute bridge above except place your feet closer than shoulder-width apart

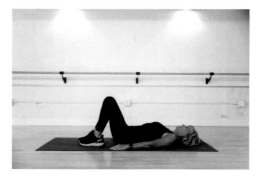

2. Slowly march in place for 5-10 seconds while your hips remain elevated by lifting one foot off the ground at a time

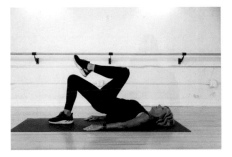

3. Focus on keeping your hips raised by driving your bottom foot into the ground as you lift the other leg

SINGLE LEG GLUTE BRIDGE

1. Perform the same setup as the glute bridge above except place your feet closer than shoulder-width apart and extend one leg

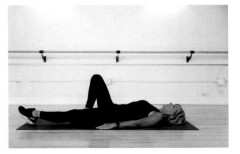

2. Drive the heel of your bent leg into the ground while pushing your hips to the ceiling until your body makes a straight line from your shoulders through your extended leg

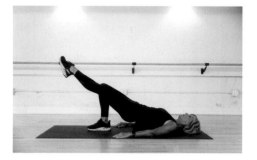

3. Keep your extended leg straight the entire time
4. Hold this position for 5-10 seconds before lowing back down

FARMER'S CARRY

1. Stand with good posture looking straight ahead while holding a heavy DB or KB in each hand

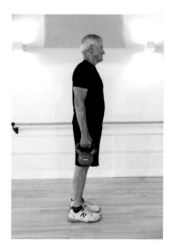

2. Your shoulders should be "down" (do not shrug them to your ears) while slightly pinching your shoulder blades together and squeezing your arms to your sides (squeeze your armpits)
3. Slightly tuck your chin straight back and brace your core (slightly contract all of your abdominal muscles)

4. Walk by taking small, light steps keeping a narrow stance

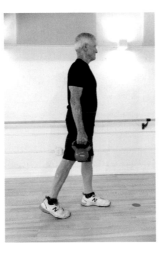

5. The weights should not swing at all while you walk

SUITCASE CARRY

1. Perform the same set up and movement as the Farmer's Carry except hold a weight in one hand only
2. Since you will only have a weight on one side the tendency will be to lean sideways as you walk so choose a weight that allows you to remain upright
3. Repeat with the weight in the other hand

STANDING TWO-ARM ROW WITH TUBING

1. Anchor or wrap a resistance tubing or band around a solid stationary object like a pole or railing at chest height
2. While holding the handles or ends of the band in each hand, step back until it is taut when your arms are outstretched, with the thumb side pointed to the ceiling

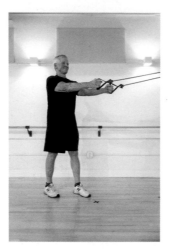

3. Assume a staggered stance position by taking a small step backwards with your opposite foot

4. Keeping an upright posture pull your elbows to your side while squeezing your shoulder blades

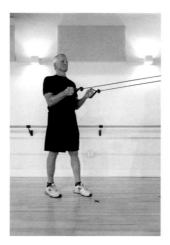

5. Your forearms should remain mostly parallel with the floor. If your hands end up by your shoulder try to focus more on driving your elbow back and keeping your hand in line with your elbow.

6. Keep a strong upright posture the entire time

STANDING SINGLE-ARM ROW WITH TUBING

1. Follow the same steps as the Two-Arm Row, but anchor the tubing so that only one end is free for you to hold

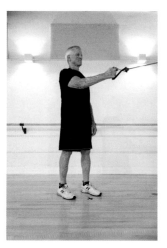

2. Hold the handle or end of the tubing in one hand and perform the movement

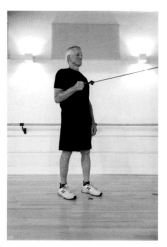

3. Do not allow your trunk to rotate during the movement

VARIATIONS:

Wide Row: From the starting position, rotate your hand so the palm side faces the floor. Instead of driving your elbow to your side, drive it out wide away from your body and keep your upper arm and forearm parallel with the ground

Half Kneeling Row: Anchor the tubing so that it is chest height when you kneel on one leg. Perform the Single Arm Row as described above. When you switch arms, switch which knee you are kneeling on. If the ground is uncomfortable, place a pillow or towel beneath your knee.

BENT OVER SINGLE-ARM DB ROW

1. While standing, hold a DB in one hand and step forward with the opposite foot to assume a staggered stance position
2. Slide your hips back, fold your trunk forward from the hips and bend your knees slightly like you would during a deadlift
3. Place your free hand on your front thigh/knee area for support while the hand holding the DB hangs toward the ground

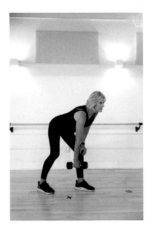

4. It is important to try to keep your trunk in a good posture so that your spine isn't rounding forward

5. From this position pull your elbow to your side to lift the weight while squeezing your shoulder blade to your spine

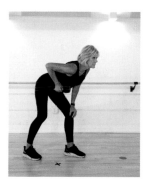

6. Do not rotate your spine while performing this movement

Tip: For some people it is easier to put their support hand on a bench or chair instead of on their front leg

BENT OVER DOUBLE-ARM DB ROW

1. Stand while holding a DB in each hand
2. Slide your hips back so that your trunk folds forward but does not round
3. Bend your knees slightly so that the DB's end up right in front of or slightly below your knees (touching or very close to them) with your palms facing your body

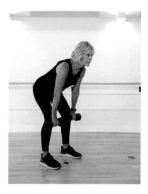

4. Pull both elbows up and out wide away from your body while squeezing both shoulder blades together

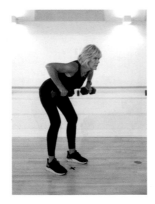

5. The inside head of the DB's should end up close to the outside edge of your shoulders

STANDING TWO-ARM CHEST PRESS WITH TUBING

1. Wrap the tubing around a pole or stair railing at chest height
2. Turn around so that your back is to the pole
3. Grab the handles in each hand and place them at chest height by your chest and shoulders with elbows away from your body
4. Step one foot forward so that the tubing pulls taut behind you

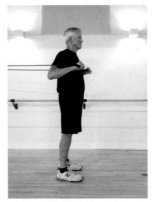

5. Push the handles away from your body until your arms are straight

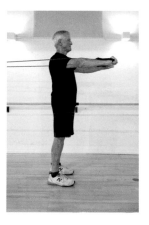

6. Slowly return to the starting position in a controlled manner
7. Remember to keep your elbows away from your body and keep your trunk in a solid upright position

STANDING SINGLE-ARM CHEST PRESS WITH TUBING

1. Anchor one end of the tubing to a pole or stair railing at chest height
2. Turn around so that your back is to the pole
3. Hold the handle in one hand and place it at chest height by your chest and shoulder with elbow away from your body

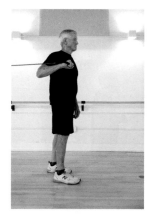

4. Walk forward until the tubing is taut and stand in a staggered stance
5. Push the handle away from you until your arm is straight

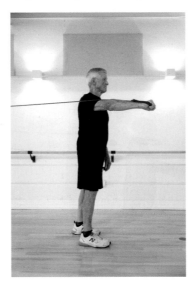

6. Slowly return to the starting position in a controlled manner
7. Maintain an upright trunk position and do not allow your trunk to twist or rotate during the movement

FULL PUSHUP

1. Get on the floor on your hands and knees with hands directly below your shoulders and knees hip-width apart
2. Straighten one leg behind you with toes flexed towards you so the ball of your foot is on the ground
3. Straighten the other leg behind you in the same manner so your hands and the balls of your feet are the only thing contacting the ground

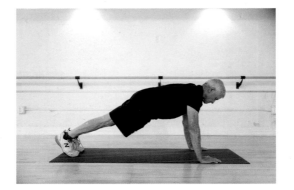

4. Lower your hips until your body makes a straight line from your shoulders to your heels and hold this position
5. Bend your elbows to lower your chest towards the ground with your elbows flaring out from your sides about 45 degrees

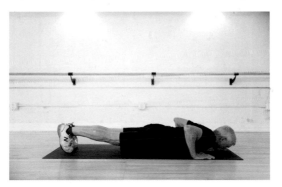

6. Lower your body as low as you can get it before pushing the floor away from you so that you return to the initial position

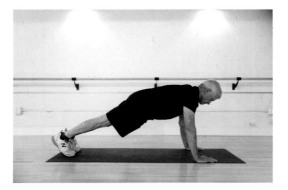

MODIFIED PUSHUP

1. Get on the floor on your hands and knees with hands directly below your shoulders and knees hip-width apart
2. Walk your hands forward so that you can lower your hips until your body makes a straight line from your shoulders to your knees

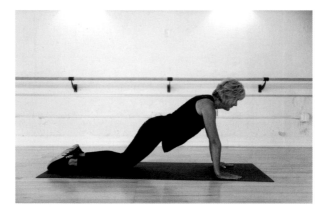

3. Bend your elbows to lower your chest towards the ground with your elbows flaring out from your sides about 45 degrees

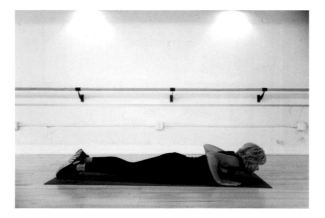

4. Lower your body as low as you can get it before pushing the floor away from you so that you return to the initial position

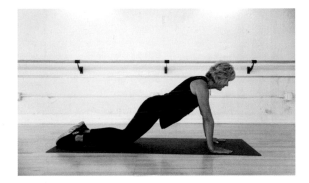

Variation: Perform the Full Pushup as described but place your hands on a stable elevated surface such as a stool or countertop. Raising the front of your body will make the pushup easier. The higher the surface, the easier it will be.

STANDING DB OVERHEAD PRESS

1. Stand with a DB in each hand
2. Place your hands next to your shoulders with palms facing you and elbows close to your sides

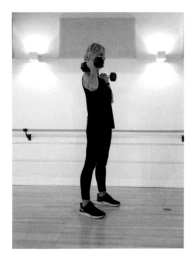

3. Push the DBs toward the ceiling until your arms are as fully extended as you can get them and then lower them to the starting position in a controlled manner

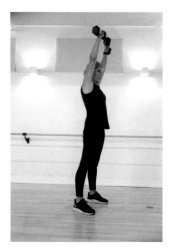

STANDING OVERHEAD PRESS WITH TUBING

1. Stand on the middle of the tubing with a handle in each hand so that there is equal length on both sides
2. Place your hands next to your shoulders with palms facing away from you and elbows close to your sides

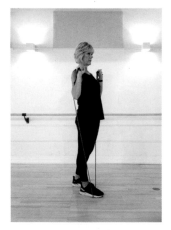

3. Push your hands towards the ceiling until your arms are as fully extended as you can get them and then lower them to the starting position in a controlled manner

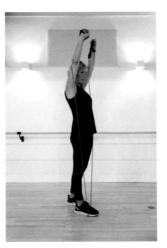

Variation: Perform the overhead press using only one arm then switch to the other arm

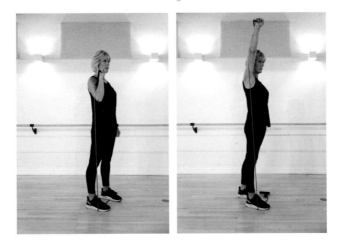

Tip: If you have shoulder problems this exercise might exacerbate them. If so, an alternative is to perform a side or a front arm raise (see below).

SIDE OR FRONT DB ARM RAISE

1. Stand with a DB in each hand with arms hanging by your sides
2. Keeping your arm mostly straight, lift the DB either in front of you or to your side until your arm is parallel with the ground
3. Lower the DB to the starting position in a controlled manner and repeat on the other side

CHAPTER 5
Exercises for Balance and Mobility

Maintaining good balance is a critical component of aging well. Falls become an increasingly serious threat with advancing age. For people in their 70s and 80s, falls are a leading cause of serious injury (including hip fracture and traumatic head injury) and accidental death. They are also the number-one reason for nursing home admissions, with many never recovering afterwards. Good balance is also important for being able to do fun things in life such as hiking, traveling, dancing, playing on the playground with grandchildren, and participating in sports, to name a few.

Like everything else, if you don't work on your balance, it will surely decline over time. Unfortunately, many people do not realize how poor their balance has gotten until they have to use it. I am often surprised by how many older adults I test who cannot even stand on one leg for longer than 5 to 10 seconds at a time. Or by how many grandparents I observe at their grandkids' ballgames that are very unsteady on the bleachers.

TAKE THIS QUICK TEST OF BALANCE

The Four Stage Balance Test is an effective quick and simple test of basic balance. Passing all four levels does not mean that your balance is as good as it needs to be but failing any of them is a good indication that it needs significant improvement. Since the four stages progress from least to most difficult the earlier you fail the worse your balance is.

Attempt to stand in each position (in the following order) for 30 seconds with your arms crossed over your chest. If you cannot hold the position for a full 30 seconds, do not move on to the next position. If you move your feet or need to take your arms off of your chest in order to maintain your balance, then the test ends. Since you may lose your balance during this test, it is best to do it with your back to the corner of a room. You may hold onto something in order to get into each position.

Stage 1 - Side By Side: Place your feet directly beside each other so that your heels and the balls of the big toes are touching.

Stage 2 - Semi-Tandem: From the side-by-side position, move one foot slightly forward so that the heel of your front foot is touching the ball of the big toe of the other foot.

Stage 3 - Full Tandem: Place one foot directly in front of the other heel to toe as if you were standing on a tightrope.

Stage 4 - Single Leg Stance: Lift one foot off the ground so it is beside your calf but without letting it touch.

BALANCE...IT'S COMPLICATED

Many people think of balance as a single thing and either you have good balance or you don't, but it is much more complicated than that. Balance is a multi-factorial concept and proper balance is dependent on multiple systems and movement strategies. These three core concepts are critical to balance training: base of support, center of gravity control, and limits of stability. Balance, at its simplest, can be considered to be control of the body's center of mass over the base of support and within a person's limits of stability.

Base of support (BOS) refers to the area beneath a person that includes every point of contact that they make with the supporting surface. These points of contact may be body parts, e.g. feet or hands, or they may include things like crutches or the chair a person is sitting in. In a standing position, a person's foot position determines their base of support. A wide foot position provides a large and stable BOS, while a narrow or single foot position creates a small and more unstable BOS. A basic progression from larger to smaller BOS is as follows:

- Wide
- Shoulder width

- Feet together (side by side)
- Semi-Tandem
- Tandem
- Single Leg

The Center of Gravity (COG), also called Center of Mass, is located just below the navel and just inside the abdominal wall for most people, although some may have an altered center of mass due to abdominal obesity or poor posture. Postural control is the ability to keep one's COG within their base of support during either static (feet do not move) or dynamic (feet move or change position) activities. If a person's COG moves outside their BOS, then they will begin to fall and will need to make quick postural adjustments in order to regain their balance. How far a person can move their COG without losing balance is called their Limits of Stability (LOS).

A person's LOS tend to decrease as they get older so that they cannot lean as far without having to take a step, but it can improve through training. The key is to move as far as possible in all directions (to their LOS) without falling. For example, during a forward lean you should lean far enough so that your heels are about to come off the ground, while during a backwards lean you should feel your toes start to come off the ground. This can be a little scary and often you will lean just a little too far and have to take a step. This is okay, as it shows that you are truly at your limits of stability. If you only stay within your comfortable range of motion, then you won't challenge yourself enough to make improvements.

Since most falls occur during dynamic movements, such as walking, it is highly recommended to challenge COG with dynamic exercises. Walking (starting and stopping), stepping (on, off, over), and changing directions/turning are all ways to challenge COG control dynamically. Increasing movement speed and complexity add to the challenge.

THE THREE POSTURAL STRATEGIES

There are three primary postural strategies that are utilized to maintain balance: Ankle, Hip, and Step. Ankle strategies (movement at the ankle joint) are used during quiet standing or when there are small perturbations and should be the first strategy that is utilized. When the ankle strategy is insufficient to maintain balance, such as during moderate perturbations, then the hip strategy (bending at the hip) is necessary. This is the second strategy that should be used. However, many older adults who are at high fall risk don't use their ankle and hip strategies like they should and instead move straight to the final strategy—the step strategy. The step strategy occurs when a person's COG moves outside their BOS. A step, in any direction, is required in order to prevent a fall from occurring. Each of these strategies can, and should, be trained so that they are utilized more effectively. Research into falls has discovered that many older adults tend to use alternative strategies such as bending their knees and reaching for support with their arms during an actual fall situation. These strategies are ineffective for reducing falls and may actually increase injury risk. For example, if a person reaches for a chair for support when they trip instead of taking a fast, powerful step, then they may be more likely to hit their head on the chair or another object.

MOBILITY. . . BALANCE AT WORK

Mobility refers to your ability to navigate within your environment—whether that be at home, work, or play. This can include walking, jogging, running, getting into and out of a chair, getting down to and up from the floor, climbing stairs, negotiating obstacles, etc. Mobility is an essential piece of overall function that is dependent on and influenced by every other functional domain. Without adequate strength and power, a person may struggle to get out of a chair or up from the floor. Without adequate cardiorespiratory endurance, a person may not be able to travel long distances. Without adequate balance, a person may not be able to navigate obstacles within their home or the community.

Since mobility is a hallmark of overall function, it is important to train mobility so you don't end up doing "the senior shuffle." This refers to the stereotypical gait pattern of a low-functioning older adult characterized by stooped posture, wider foot position, smaller strides, more side to side movement, and slower walking speed in general. Slow gait speed is a hallmark sign of overall functional impairment that predicts future disability. It is also one of the earliest signs that the gait cycle is beginning to become impaired.

There are many factors that can impair the gait cycle including pain, cognitive function, orthopedic conditions, and neurological conditions. In many cases, the gait pattern can improve considerably with proper exercise training, especially if the changes are primarily due to deconditioning. However, in some cases there are underlying factors that need to be corrected or addressed because these will continue to affect the gait cycle. For example, a person with severe osteoarthritis who has no cartilage left in their knee will not be likely to normalize their gait pattern through exercise training alone. Exercise, in the absence of a total joint replacement, will do very little to minimize the pain and immobility associated with this condition.

The primary goal of mobility training is to make the gait flexible and adaptable so that you are able to easily negotiate environmental challenges such as a sloped floor/ground, uneven surfaces (grass, rocks), unstable surfaces (slippery spots), obstacles (curbs, cones, etc.), moving in different directions (forward, backward, lateral), directional changes, and the need to accelerate or decelerate quickly. In order to accomplish this, a wide variety of mobility exercises must be used that will "force" the body to move in lots of different ways that either emphasize or accentuate normal gait mechanics. For example, individuals tend to use quicker strides because they do not want to be in single limb support, since that requires a greater degree of balance. Challenging clients to take very slow steps with a prolonged single stance phase will improve this one aspect of their gait mechanics.

BALANCE AND FALL PREVENTION

Falls are due to a number of internal and external factors. Internal factors that increase fall risk include a history of falls, age, living alone, certain medications, impaired mobility and gait, sedentary behavior, visual impairments, poor lower extremity strength, and fear of falling (Todd 2004). External risk factors include environmental hazards (poor lighting, slippery floors, uneven surfaces, etc.); improper footwear and clothing; and the use of walking aids or assistive devices (Todd 2004). Exercise has been identified as the best single intervention to prevent falls in older adults, with up to 42 percent of falls being preventable by a well-designed exercise program (Todd 2004; Gillespie et al 2009). Other effective interventions include home safety modifications, medication reduction or substitution (especially psychoactive or CNS depressant medications), reducing fear of falling, and surgery to correct cataracts.

All of the systems responsible for proper balance can improve with proper training, which should lead to a reduction in fall risk and, ultimately, a reduction in fall prevalence. Determining which systems are deficient for an individual is a critical step in developing an effective training program. The optimal balance training approach may differ widely from person to person, but there are a number of broad recommendations that have been culled from the research.

KEY BALANCE TRAINING RECOMMENDATIONS

Recommendation 1. Exercise must provide a moderate or high challenge to balance. Programs that do not challenge balance are not effective in preventing falls. Balance should be challenged in three ways: 1) Reducing base of support; 2) Movement of the center of gravity; and 3) Reducing the need for upper limb support during standing exercise.

Recommendation 2. Exercise must be of a sufficient dose to have an effect. At least 2 hours per week of exercise for a 6-month period appears to be sufficient.

Recommendation 3. Ongoing exercise is necessary. Balance improvements are lost quickly upon the cessation of exercise.

Recommendation 4. Falls prevention exercise should be targeted at the general community as well as those at high risk for falls.

Recommendation 5. Falls prevention exercise may be undertaken in a group or home-based setting.

Recommendation 6. Walking training may be included in addition to balance training, but high-risk individuals should not be prescribed brisk walking programs. Walking training is not a crucial feature of effective falls prevention programs. Therefore, walking should only be included if it does not infringe upon or decrease the effects of the balance training.

Recommendation 7. Strength training may be included in addition to balance training. Strength training is not a crucial aspect of falls prevention programs but may be included due to its many benefits for older populations.

Recommendation 8. Exercise providers should make referrals for other risk factors to be addressed. As part of a comprehensive approach to falls reduction, evidence-based interventions targeting specific risk factors should be provided by appropriate health professionals.

The following exercises will challenge your balance and mobility in different ways, some of which may be difficult and some of which may be easy. The goal is to choose movements that are challenging but doable. Since performing balance exercises is somewhat risky, it is okay to if you need to use a sturdy object, like a piece of furniture or a handrail, to provide some assistance but, over time, try to gradually decrease your dependence on it.

BALANCE AND MOBILITY EXERCISES

FOUR STAGE BALANCE

This is a progressive balance challenge that moves from easiest to most difficult. Start with the easiest position and when you can hold that position for 30 seconds or more move on to the next hardest position. Always stand close to a solid, stable object that you can use for balance if needed. It is good to practice this both with and without shoes.

1. Stand with a good upright posture with arms crossed over your chest while looking straight ahead (it helps to focus on a solid object directly in front of you at eye height)
2. Position 1: Place feet side-by-side so that heels and balls of the big toes touch

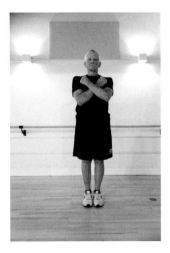

3. Position 2: Move one foot slightly forward so that the heel of the front foot touches the ball of the big toe of the back foot (called the "Semi-Tandem" position)

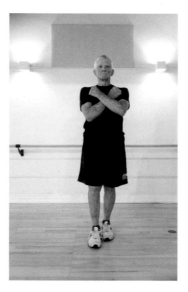

4. Position 3: Place one foot directly in front of the other foot so that the heel of the front foot touches the toes of the back foot as if you were walking a tight rope (called the "Full Tandem" position)

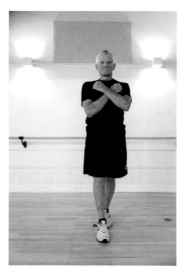

5. Position 4: Raise one foot off the ground so that it is beside, but not touching, the calf of the stance leg (called the "Single Leg Stance" position)

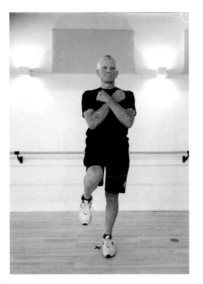

Tip: Use "Short Foot" to help you balance. Short Foot is a simple strategy that can improve your balance. Start by finding your foot "tripod" which is the heel, ball of the big toe, and ball of the pinky toe. Shift your weight around so that it is distributed equally between these three points of contact. Next, lift and spread your toes and firmly "grab" the floor with your toes (just like you would with your hand). When you do so you should feel the arch of your foot "lift". Maintain this short foot position while you attempt the Four Stage Balance exercise. It is also helpful to use during squats and deadlifts.

SINGLE LEG STANCE WITH HEAD TURNS

Once you've mastered the Single Leg Stance (meaning you can hold it for 30 seconds or longer) then try this advanced version.

1. Assume the Single Leg Stance position as described earlier

2. While your leg is lifted, slowly turn your head to the right and to the left, shifting your gaze with your head movement

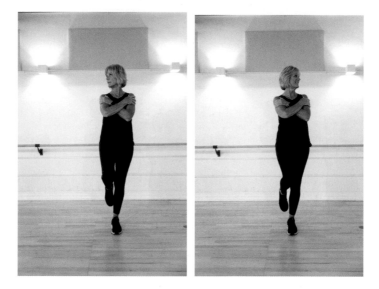

3. You may need to practice while lightly holding onto an object for balance and then gradually moving to an arms crossed position

ANKLE SWAY

This is a very small, but important movement that involves moving forward and backward ONLY using your ankles. The distance we can lead forward and backward from the ankle is called our "Sway Envelope" and it is a good indicator of fall risk.

1. Stand in an upright posture with feet directly beside one another (you may first try this in a shoulder-width position but then try to make your stance more narrow)
2. Moving ONLY about the ankles lean forward as far as you can go. You should feel your toes digging into the ground and your heels wanting to come off the ground.

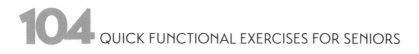

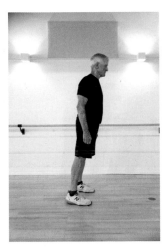

3. Then lean backwards as far as you can you. You should feel your weight shift onto your heels and your toes wanting to come off the ground.

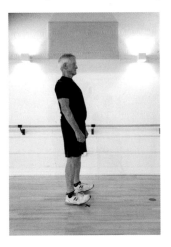

4. Continue slowly cycling between a forward lean and a backward lean
5. The key is to NOT bend at the hips, which is the natural inclination
6. Be prepared to take a step either forward or backward as you will likely lean a little too far and start to fall. This is actually a good thing as you must challenge yourself if you are going to improve.

CLOCK TOUCHES

1. Stand in an upright posture with feet close together.
2. Imagine that you are standing in the middle of a big clock face with all of the numbers (1-12) circling you (12 directly in front; 3 directly to your right, etc.)
3. Reach one foot out towards the 12 as far as you can and lightly touch the floor while keeping your weight on your stance leg

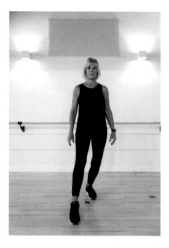

4. Return to the starting position and repeat for the 1:00 position, then 2:00 position, and so on until you reach 6:00

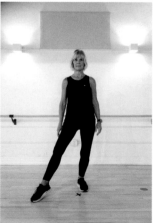

5. Repeat with the other leg starting at 12:00 but moving counter-clockwise to 11:00, 10:00, and so on until you reach 6:00
6. It is important to reach as far in each direction as you can without losing your balance

TANDEM WALK (AKA "TIGHTROPE WALK")

1. Start in a Full Tandem Position with one foot directly in front of the other, with the heel of the front foot touching the toes of the back foot
2. Walk forward by placing your back foot directly in front of your front foot so your heel touches your toes

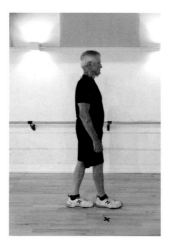

3. Continue alternating feet
4. Try to look straight ahead at an object instead of looking down at your feet

TANDEM MARCH

1. Perform the Tandem Walk as described above but with each step, lift your knee in front of you (like you were marching) before placing it back down in front of the other

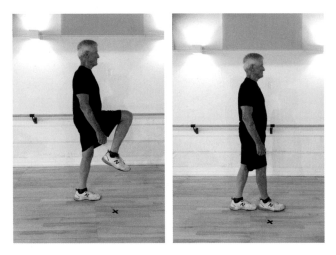

BRAIDED WALK OR MARCH

Perform the Tandem Walk or March as described but instead of placing one foot directly in front of the other, cross it over the other as if you were stepping over a line instead of stepping on the line

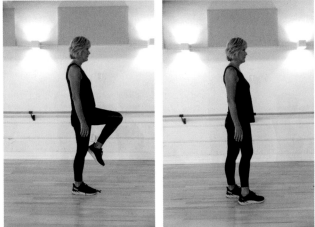

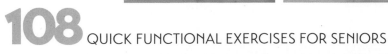

STRAIGHT LEG MARCH (AKA "MILITARY MARCH")

March forward but instead of bending your knee keep your leg straight as you raise it up and down

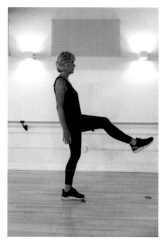

HEEL WALK

1. From a normal standing position pull your toes towards your shins so only your heels are in contact with the floor

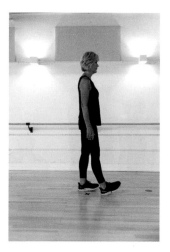

2. Take small steps forward while keeping your toes off of the ground at all times
3. This will look rather awkward as you will need to keep your knees relatively straight while you are walking

TOE WALK

1. From a normal standing position raise up on the balls of your feel so that your heels are off the ground as high as they will go

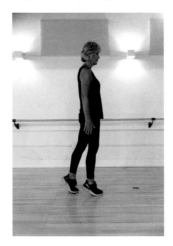

2. Walk forward while staying on the balls of your feet and keeping your heels off the ground

WALK THE RAILS

1. Assume a wide stance position as if you had each foot on a railroad track
2. Slightly bend at your knees as you walk forward keeping your feet wide apart as all times just as if you were walking down the railroad track

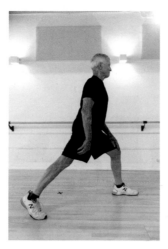

MARCH IN PLACE WITH HEAD TURNS

1. From a standing position begin marching in place by alternately raising one knee in front of your body at a time to hip height
2. Swing your bent arms as you normally would when you are marching or walking with opposite hand and knee coming forward
3. Match the cadence of your marching by alternately turning your head to the same side as the knee that you lift

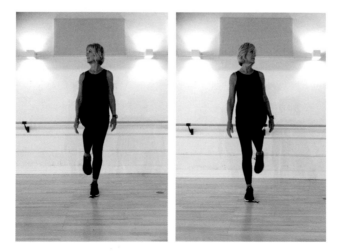

4. Maintain a slow steady rhythm at first and then gradually speed up as you are able
5. It is important to synchronize the head turns with the knee lifts

WALKING WITH HEAD TURNS

1. Walk straight ahead using confident strides swinging your bent arms as you normally would when walking with opposite hand and foot coming forward
2. Match the cadence of your stepping by alternately turning your head to the same side as the foot you are stepping forward with (e.g. look to the right when you step forward with your right foot)

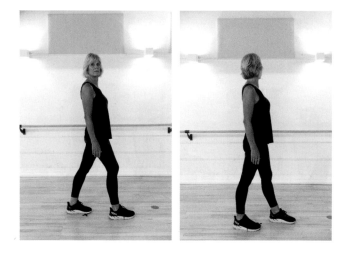

3. Your rhythm should be steady using a normal walking pattern
4. Your path should be straight ahead with veering to the right or left
5. Your head turns and stepping should be synchronized

CARIOCHE (AKA "GRAPEVINE")

1. This is a lateral movement that requires you to cross your feet
2. Start in a normal standing position

3. Move to the left by stepping your right foot over your left foot

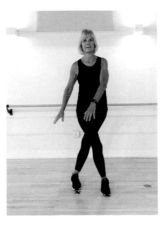

4. Continue moving left by stepping your right foot behind your left foot

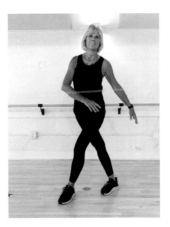

5. Continue repeating this pattern of stepping your right foot in front of and then behind your left foot
6. Reverse the pattern to move to the right
7. Start slowly and then once you get the hang of it gradually increase your speed until it becomes a faster and more "athletic" type of movement
8. A faster movement will require you to turn your hips one way while you turn your upper body in the opposite direction and to stay up on the balls of your feet more

Advanced Variations for Walks and Marches:
   Eyes Closed: Close your eyes while performing
   Backwards: Perform by walking backwards
   Eyes Closed Backwards: Close your eyes while walking backwards
   Head Turns: Turn your head to the right when you step forward with the right foot and turn your head to the left when you step forward with the left foot

HOPSCOTCH
Yes, this is just like the game you probably played as a kid but without having to draw squares on the ground.

1.   Start with feet shoulder-width apart

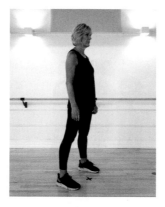

2.   Hop onto your right leg with the left leg lifted off the ground

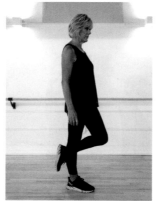

3. Hop back into a shoulder-width stance

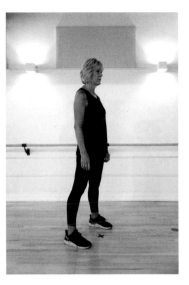

4. Hop onto the left leg with the right leg lifted off the ground

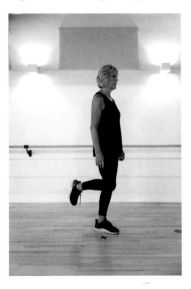

5. Hop back into a shoulder-width stance

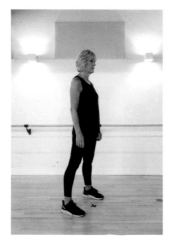

6. Repeat this sequence for 10-15 seconds
7. You may do this in place or move forward with each hop just like you do in Hopscotch

BUNNY HOPS

1. Start in a standing position with feet shoulder-width apart
2. Crouch down slightly with your arms bent or by your side

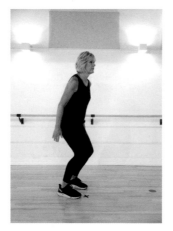

3. Hop forward about 6-12 inches making sure both feet move together and land softly

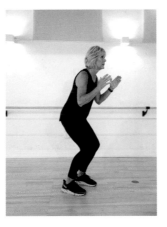

4. Pause to make sure you are well-balanced and hop forward again
5. Drive your arms forward when you jump and focus on jumping forward rather than up
6. Gradually increase the distance you are jumping as you are able

LINE HOPS

1. Try to find a place where there is a line or small crack on the floor
2. Stand directly behind the line/crack with toes almost touching it
3. Keeping soft knees and bending slightly at the hips, hop forward over the line/crack and then quickly hop backwards over the line to return to the starting position
4. Continue hopping forwards and backwards over the line
5. Start slowly and then gradually speed up as fast as you are able
6. Try to stay on the balls of your feet as much as possible
7. Hop for 10-15 seconds

Line Hop Variation: Stand beside the line instead of behind it and jump sideways (right and left) over the line as quickly as you can

FEET SWITCHES

1. Try to find a place where there is a line or small crack on the floor
2. Stand straddling the line with your right foot over the line and left foot behind the line a little narrower than shoulder-width apart
3. Your arms should be bent (as if running) with the left arm in front of your shoulder and right arm behind your shoulder

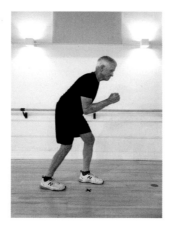

4. Switch feet positions by moving both feet and arms at the same time so now the other foot is in front and the other foot is behind the line
5. Your arms will also have changed positions
6. Continue doing this as quickly as possible for 10-15 seconds

CHAPTER 6
Core and Posture Exercises

The core/trunk musculature is the connection between the upper and lower body and is one of the hidden keys to good posture and better function. These muscles form a corset, or weight belt, around your spine to keep it safe during loaded activities such as lifting, carrying, reaching, and twisting. These muscles connect the ribs, pelvis (hips), and spine (vertebrae). It is important to build stability in all directions in the core muscles in a way that will enable movement while reducing potentially dangerous loads on the spine. A core that is stable is one that keeps the spine in what is called a neutral position during daily, work-related, and sports movements. It is the neutral spine position that keeps the back safe during activities. Traditionally, many abdominal exercises are dynamic movements such as crunches, sit-ups, and leg raises. These types of movements require the spine to flex and bend in different directions, which creates potentially dangerous loads because they take the spine out of the neutral position. While many people can perform these exercises without too much trouble, older spines tend to be less forgiving, making them more susceptible to injury—especially those with degenerative changes in their spine.

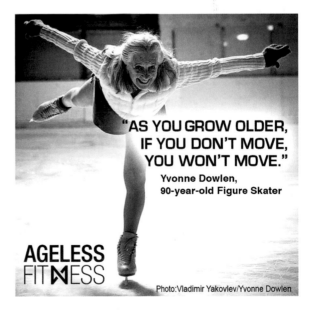

"AS YOU GROW OLDER, IF YOU DON'T MOVE, YOU WON'T MOVE."

Yvonne Dowlen,
90-year-old Figure Skater

AGELESS FITNESS

Photo: Vladimir Yakovlev/Yvonne Dowlen

Therefore, effective core training focuses on keeping the spine in the same neutral position while performing loaded movements such as weight-lifting exercises. This is accomplished by contracting all of the core muscles simultaneously—a technique called bracing—to prevent movement rather than create movement. These exercises can challenge the core in either the sagittal plane (bending forwards or backwards), frontal plane (bending sideways), and/or transverse plane (twisting or rotating). Exercises such as front planks (sagittal plane), side planks (frontal plane), and shoulder-tap planks (transverse plane) are good examples of core stability exercises.

CORE MUSCLES

RECTUS ABDOMINIS
These are your front set of muscles known as your "six-pack" muscles. They run vertically to connect the front of your ribs to the front of your pelvis. These muscles help you flex your spine forward, tense the front wall of the stomach, and help with compression of the midsection.

OBLIQUES
There are two sets of oblique muscles (internal and external) on either side of your body. They connect the front and side of the lower half of ribs to your pelvis in a criss-cross ("X") pattern. They play a key role in side-bending and trunk rotation while assisting to stabilize the core.

TRANSVERSE ABDOMINIS
This is the deepest abdominal muscle that runs sideways encircling your waist and connecting to your spine in the back and to the linea alba (the line of connective tissue you may see in between the six-pack muscles). It may be the most important muscle overall because it holds your internal organs in place and stabilizes the spine and pelvis even before you move your arms or legs. It also assists with trunk rotation. Inadequate activation of this muscle is associated with low back pain and lumbar instability.

SPINAL EXTENSORS

There are several different types of muscles that run up and down your spine vertically. They assist with all sorts of spinal movements, help to stabilize and compress the spine during loading, and are especially important in extension (arching your back).

OTHER

Many other muscles that attach to the spine and hips contribute to core stability including the quadratus lumborum (QL), pelvic floor, diaphragm, and latissimus dorsi ("lats"). Engaging these muscles in addition to the ones listed above can be helpful for keeping the spine stiff and safe.

THREE KEY STRATEGIES

There are three key strategies you will need to learn: 1) How to find neutral spine; 2) How to brace using your core muscles; and 3) How to hip hinge properly. These strategies will help you learn how to move better and safer and will allow you to get stronger while keeping your spine protected. These are especially important if you already have lower back pain, poor posture, or other issues related to your spine.

1. <u>How to Find Neutral Spine</u>: In a standing position, stand tall and perform several posterior and anterior pelvic tilts without changing your upper trunk position. Think of your hips like a cup. For an anterior pelvic tilt, imagine pouring the cup out in front of you by moving your bottom backwards (no bending at the waist). For a posterior pelvic tilt, empty the cup out behind you by tucking your tail underneath you. Do this several times to find the "happy place" in between those two positions that feels the most comfortable. Your pelvis should be fairly level at this point, which is going to be your neutral spine position. Relax and move around a bit before returning to the standing position and repeating the sequence. Since the goal is to be able to find the neutral spine position while you are performing exercises, then it is necessary to keep practicing this. It is often helpful to find neutral spine in the seated and quadruped (on your hands and knees) positions.

2. <u>How to Brace</u>: Bracing the trunk requires activation of all of the core musculature (rectus abdominis, transverse abdominis, internal obliques, external obliques, erector spinae, etc.). The challenge is that many people have a difficult time activating these muscles. There are several techniques that can be helpful:

   - Cough and feel the core muscles tense
   - Pretend that someone is punching you in the stomach and tense up accordingly
   - Use your fingers to "grab" or push into your core muscles (front and sides). Do not do this lightly. The goal is for it to be somewhat uncomfortable so that you tense your muscles against your fingers.
   - Stand tall in neutral spine with feet just outside of shoulder-width apart to create a strong base. Stay tall and rigid like a statue. Have someone apply pressure to your shoulder from the side with one hand (as if they were going to push you over), starting lightly and gradually increasing the force. Resist their pushing and remain stiff. You should feel this activating the core muscles on the side they are pushing from and in the front. You can use your hand to "grab" or "poke" those activated muscles so that you can better feel what is happening. Repeat on the other side. Then do the same thing, pushing you from the front or from the back, but stagger your stance with one foot slightly ahead of the other to keep it from pushing you over easily. Remember that you only need enough pushing force to feel those muscles activate. Do not have them apply so much force that it pushes you out of neutral spine.

Once you get a good feel for these muscles, try to contract them on your own while in a neutral spine position. When you do so, your upper body should not move or change position. Many people flex their front muscles so much that it pulls them forward and out of spinal neutral. So stay tall while you contract them. When bracing, continue to breathe shallowly through your chest. Full, deep "belly" breaths will not be possible without relaxing your core muscles because the diaphragm will not be able to draw downwards. The focus, instead, will be on expansion of the rib cage for breathing. Only under very heavy loading, such as heavy squats or deadlifts, is a Valsalva (i.e. breath holding) technique appropriate. This helps to create a lot of intra-abdominal pressure but should only be performed during a single repetition. Breathe in and hold your breath to perform the heavy repetition. Breathe out when the repetition is completed and breathe in again for the next repetition. Never hold your breath continuously through multiple repetitions, as this can cause lightheadedness or even unconsciousness.

3. How to Hip Hinge: The hip hinge involves bending forwards and backwards at the hip while maintaining spinal neutral through proper bracing. It is very difficult for some individuals to separate bending forward at the hips from bending forward with the spine. Think of your hips as a doorframe and your spine as the door. When a door swings from its hinges it doesn't bend at all, as the movement only comes from the hinge. Likewise, during a proper hip hinge movement, the spine does not bend but merely rotates on the hips (like a door hinge). This movement is necessary for performing a deadlift exercise as well as performing tasks in daily life, such as lifting something from the floor. When you bend from the spine when you lean over (i.e. you round your back), you put the back in a potentially unsafe position when lifting loads. So, it is better to learn how to perform a proper hip hinge movement pattern. Several cues can be helpful when learning the hip hinge.
    a. Think of "shutting the file cabinet drawer" behind you with your bottom. Stand with your back to a wall a few inches away so that your bottom touches the wall when you move it backwards.
    b. Instead of leaning over, simply slide your hips backwards so that your trunk naturally falls over like a tower.
    c. Add a resistance band around your hips pulling them backwards (light resistance) while you perform the "shut the drawer" maneuver.
    d. Place a dowel rod or PVC pipe along your spine so that it touches the back of your head, the top of your spine, and your tailbone while you perform the "shut the drawer" maneuver. All three points should remain in contact with the rod during the movement.
    e. Try the "shortstop position" by sliding your hands down your thighs until they rest just above the knees. Adjust your spinal position to neutral if you have flexed or extended the spine by using your pelvic tilt.

f. Keep your head in alignment with your spine at all times. For example, when you lean forward, do not try to keep your head up by arching your neck. Instead, keep it in the same position on your shoulders the entire time.

g. Use a mirror so you can see your form while you hip hinge. Notice any change in your spine position while you move. It is helpful to move slowly.

During a hip hinge movement, the amount of hip flexion or forward bending you can achieve will be limited mainly by your flexibility. Only lean forward to the point where you experience tightness in your hamstrings and glutes while maintaining spinal neutral and then stop. This becomes your maximal hip hinge ability because any more forward bending will need to come from spinal flexion, which is to be avoided. Once you feel like you can perform a proper hip hinge, repeatedly add resistance via a resistance band or kettlebell. Having a little bit of resistance in your hands can help you to better "feel" the movement pattern.

BUILD ISOMETRIC ENDURANCE FIRST

Since core stability exercises should challenge the trunk musculature without deviating from spinal neutral; this means the exercises should be isometric (muscle contraction without joint movement) and the first goal is to build isometric endurance. This is typically accomplished by holding a position for anywhere from 10 to 60 seconds. Once endurance is established, then you can progress to heavier loading to build strength or faster movements to develop power. Here are some isometric exercises that are effective for building core endurance.

1. Bird Dog – From a quadruped position, slowly extend arm or extend leg or extend opposite arm and leg (transverse)
2. Dead Bug – Lie on back with arms extended towards ceiling and bent legs extended towards ceiling (quadruped position but on your back). Extend one arm over head and return to the start. Extend a leg and return to the start. Extend opposite arm and leg and return to the start. (transverse)

3. Planks – There are many variations of the plank position which can accommodate users with varying abilities and challenge multiple planes of movement.
   a. Front Plank (sagittal)
      i. Low Front Plank – performed prone on elbow(s)
      ii. High Front Plank – performed prone on hand(s)
      iii. Elevated Front Plank – performed prone with hands/elbows on an elevated surface such as a bench, table, or wall
      iv. Modified Front Plank – performed prone with knees on ground instead of toes/feet
      v. Reverse Plank – performed in supine typically with feet elevated onto a bench or chair
   b. Side Plank – performed on one elbow (low plank) or hand (high plank) with body turned to the side (frontal)
   c. Shoulder-Tap Plank – from the high plank position, slowly touch one hand to the opposite shoulder, return to start position, and repeat with the other hand (transverse)
   d. Rolling Plank – from the low or high plank position, "roll" into a side plank position, return to the start, and roll to a side plank position on the other side (sagittal, frontal, and transverse)
4. Glute Bridges
   a. Double-leg (sagittal)
   b. Single-leg (transverse)
5. Pallof Press – Hold cable or tubing in both hands in front of the navel with arms bent. Resistance should be pulling laterally (anchored beside you). (transverse)
   a. Add sideways stepping to make it a dynamic exercise

Many standard resistance exercises can also be performed in a manner that requires a great deal of trunk stability. This is an effective and efficient way to build endurance and strength in the trunk musculature and has many direct functional applications. Movements such as presses and rows, if performed without external support, will automatically require trunk stability. These can be performed in standing, half-kneeling, and kneeling positions with bands/tubing, cables, and free weights (depending on the body position and movement). Using either bilateral (both arms) or unilateral (single-arm) movements will also change the challenge to the trunk musculature. Horizontal presses will predominantly activate the anterior chain musculature (e.g. rectus abdominis), while horizontal rows will predominantly active the posterior chain musculature (e.g. erector spinae). It is important to include a wide variety of core stability exercises so that all three planes are challenged consistently in a program.

JOINT MOBILITY AND FLEXIBILITY

Having good posture and moving well is also dependent, to some degree, on how mobile and flexible we are or, conversely, how inflexible we are. We don't need to have the bendiness of a gymnast, but when we start moving like Frankenstein that's a problem. Unfortunately, most people's joints become less and less able to move freely as they get older, usually for one of three reasons. First, the biological process of aging leads to significant losses in collagen (which is what gives our muscles and joints their flexibility). Second, we spend lots of time in poor postures (typically stooped forward over a book, phone, or computer), which creates chronic negative changes in our muscle balance. And third, we simply don't work on our flexibility enough. It is really the third reason that has the biggest impact, since people who continue to work on being flexible maintain most, if not all, of their joint range of motion as they get older. Deficits in flexibility with advancing age have been identified as contributing to the development of a number of acute and chronic conditions including postural deviations (kyphosis, forward head, rounded shoulders), lower back pain, and rotator cuff tendinitis.

There are several areas of the body that warrant special attention—the ankles, hips, and thoracic spine (the section of your spine located just above to a couple inches below your shoulder blades). These three areas combined can have a significant impact on both posture and overall function when their mobility is lost. Since the body is an interconnected system, poor mobility in one area tends to lead to issues in other areas. For example, knee pain may often develop due to a lack of mobility at either the ankles or hips or both. The knee is a hinge joint, meaning that it really only wants to move primarily front to back, which is called flexion and extension. But since it is sandwiched in between the ankle and knee, it is often forced to bend in other directions when they aren't able to move like they should which, over time, can lead to knee discomfort, pain, and even injury. Knee pain can then cause you to start moving differently (even when you don't realize it) in order to minimize the pain. This can create a chain reaction, which could contribute to poor posture, low back pain, and other movement problems. It is beneficial, therefore, to spend some time performing stretching and mobility exercises, especially for these three key areas of the body.

Ankle Dorsiflexion: Lack of ankle dorsiflexion can significantly impact squatting/sitting and gait patterns and can increase fall risk. Limited dorsiflexion (how far your knee will go past your toe or how far you can pull your toes back toward your shin) can be due to soft tissue inflexibility (calf tightness), improper movement of the ankle joint, or a combination of the two. A helpful way to evaluate ankle dorsiflexion is to assume a half-kneeling position without shoes on with the toes touching a wall. Drive your front knee forward as far as you can go without your heel coming off of the ground. At a minimum, you should be able to get your knee to touch the wall in this position but, ideally, you should still be able to touch the wall when your foot is 1 to 2 inches away from the wall so that your knee goes past your toes. If you cannot, then this indicates limited dorsiflexion. While you are performing this test, notice where you feel the limitation. Is it a tight stretch in the calf muscle (back of your shin) or a discomfort (like a pinching feeling) in the front of the ankle? If you say the calf muscle, then traditional calf stretches and foam rolling will be helpful. However, if you say discomfort in the front of the ankle, then you probably have an issue in the ankle itself. Individuals that have severely or repeatedly "rolled" their ankle when they were younger are more likely to have joint ankle issues due to the build-up of scar tissue.

To correct the joint ankle limitation, place a strong super band around your ankle while your foot is propped up on a small stool or box and the other foot is on the ground. The band should be anchored behind you (around a pole or under a heavy weight) at a slightly downward angle and stretched to provide a significant amount of resistance. From this position, bend your front knee a little more and drive your knee forward (just like you did on the test) to perform bent-knee calf stretches. Track you knee outwards slightly toward your second toe (beside their pinky toe). Hold that position for 3 to 5 seconds, relax and repeat for a total of 10 repetitions. For best results, perform 2 to 3 sets daily. If performed correctly, you should feel more of a stretch in the calf and less discomfort in the front of the ankle, but it may take a little time to restore the proper motion.

As ankle dorsiflexion improves, it is important to load it in functional positions such as during squatting. This will help your body learn how to use that new-found range of motion in a functional pattern. The body will have made compensations for the lack of ankle dorsiflexion and will need to re-learn proper muscle activation patterns in order to fully take advantage of this improvement.

Hip Mobility: The hips are a big, important structure for almost anything we do because they are home to some of the largest muscle groups in the body such as the glutes, hamstrings, and quadriceps. Proper hip mobility is required for many functional activities, and when it is lacking it can create issues all along the kinetic chain (especially for the ankles, knees, and lower back) which may lead to acute or chronic pain. It is also a factor in performing, or as a pre-requisite for performing, many exercises appropriately such as squats, deadlifts, and lunges. Since the hips move in many different directions such as frontwards/backwards (flexion/extension), apart and together (abduction/adduction), and turning in and out (internal/external rotation), a variety of mobility exercises are recommended that address each of these directions.

TOE TOUCH SCREEN

A combination of hamstring (back of the thighs) and glute inflexibility tends to be a common issue among older adults that can limit their ability to lean forward, squat, deadlift and move well, in general. A quick measure of these can be accomplished via the Toe Touch Screen.

For this test, stand side by side so that your feet touch (heels and balls of the big toes). Without bending your knees, breathe in and then slowly bend forward while you exhale so that your fingers reach for your toes. Relax your back so that it rounds forward but do not bend your knees. Get as close to your toes as possible. Pause and then stand up again.

Ideally, you should be able to reach the tops of your toes or the floor. If you are able to get within 1-2 inches then your flexibility needs a little work but is pretty good overall. The further away you get from this ideal indicates worsening flexibility of these muscles which may contribute to moving poorly. Since this assessment allows you to round your spine forward then it doesn't just target the hips but the entire back as well. Being very flexible in the spine may allow you to reach your toes even though your hamstrings and glutes may still be overly tight.

Thoracic Spine Mobility: A lack of mobility in the thoracic spine can lead to all sorts of common issues such as postural deviations, decreased shoulder mobility, inability to turn your trunk fully, compensation patterns, and a general decrease in upper-body function. The most common postural deviation is kyphosis (forward flexion—like a small humpback position), which is often accompanied by a forward-head position (often called "turtle head"). This is primarily due to the fact that we tend to spend a lot of time in a kyphotic, forward-head position while working on a computer, using our phone, or reading. Therefore, most people become limited in thoracic extension and rotation at the same time. Thoracic motion is also closely linked to shoulder mobility. A lack of shoulder mobility (e.g. you can't reach straight over your head with both arms) is often due to a combination of shoulder and thoracic spine tightness.

TEST OF THORACIC MOBILITY

For this test, you will need a chair, dowel (or broom handle or yard stick), and a bed pillow.

Sit upright in a sturdy flat chair (like a dining room chair) and scoot toward the front. Your knees should be bent at 90 degrees with your feet together flat on the floor. Place a folded pillow between your knees and squeeze it lightly. Place the dowel across your collarbones at the base of your neck and cross your arms to hold it in place. Turn your head and shoulders as far to the left as possible without moving your hips or bottom (squeezing the pillow with your knees helps to prevent your hips and legs from moving). Have someone note how far you were able to turn. Relax and return to center. Repeat the process, turning to your right.

Scoring: You should be able to turn to about 45 degrees or more to each side. If either or both sides do not reach 45 degrees, you should work on your thoracic mobility by doing extension and rotation exercises daily.

Since spinal extension and rotation are inter-dependent in the thoracic spine, it is important to work on both of these. However, if you have pre-existing spinal conditions such as degenerative discs, spinal fusions, or osteoporosis, do these with caution or consult either a physician or physical therapist before doing them.

CORE AND POSTURE EXERCISES

Plank exercises are great for developing core strength and stability and improving posture. They differ from many traditional exercises because they require you to hold a position rather than moving through a range of motion. The position should be held for about 10-15 seconds at a time and then relaxing for about 5-10 seconds before performing the next one.

The most common mistake many people make is holding their breath while they are holding their position. It will be more difficult to breathe while holding a plank position because you have to contract all of your core muscles. This means your diaphragm doesn't have anywhere to go. So, while performing a plank focus on shallow breaths through your upper chest (rather than belly breathing) so that you don't relax your core muscles.

FRONT PLANK

1. Lie face down on the floor with your forearms propped under your shoulders and toes pulled towards your body
2. Your elbows should be directly under your shoulders making a 90-degree angle with your forearms
3. In one motion lift your entire body so that if makes a straight line from your shoulders to your heels while pushing your forearms into the ground

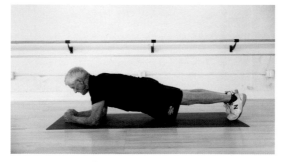

4. The only parts contacting the ground should be your forearms/elbows and the balls of your feet
5. Avoid pushing your hips too high so that your body is not in a straight line

6. You will need to contract your abdominal and buttock muscles to maintain a rigid position

HIGH PLANK

1. Get on the floor on your hands and knees with hands directly below your shoulders and knees hip-width apart
2. Straighten one leg behind you with toes flexed towards you so the ball of your foot is on the ground
3. Straighten the other leg behind you in the same manner so your hands and the balls of your feet are the only thing contacting the ground
4. Lower your hips until your body makes a straight line from your shoulders to your heels and hold this position

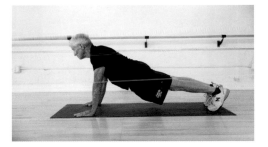

HIGH PLANK WITH SHOULDER TAPS

1. Assume a high plank position as described above but move your hands to just within shoulder-width and spread out your feet to just outside of hip-width

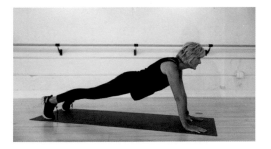

2. While holding this position touch your right shoulder with your left hand in a slow and controlled manner and then place it back on the ground in the same spot

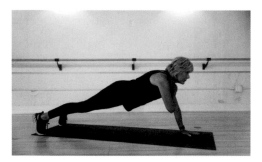

3. Repeat by touching your left shoulder with your right hand in the same manner
4. Try to maintain the same body position (no twisting or bending) while you do this

Tip: If doing this on the floor is too difficult, then elevate the front part of your body by placing your forearms or hands on a stable bench, chair or countertop. The higher the surface the easier the exercise will be.

SIDE PLANK

1. Lie on your side with your elbow and forearm propped directly under your bottom shoulder and your top foot placed just in front of your bottom foot

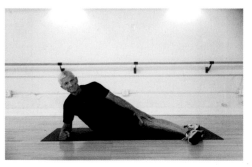

2. Push your elbow and feet into the ground while pushing the top side of your hip towards the ceiling until your body is in a straight-line position from head to feet

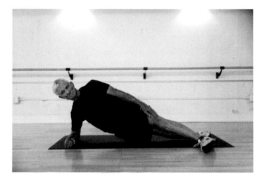

3. Hold this position

REVERSE PLANK

1. Lie on your back with your heels propped up on a step or small stool and your hands by your side

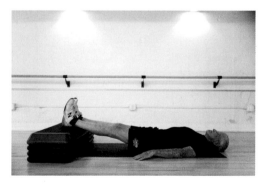

2. Place a small pillow or towel under your head if it is too uncomfortable to place it on the ground

3. Drive your heels into the step while pushing your hips toward the ceiling until your body is in straight-line position from shoulders to feet and hold this position

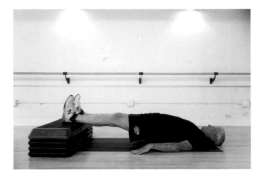

4. Avoid pressing the back of your head into the ground but, rather, let the weight of your body fall on the back of your shoulders

T-PLANK ROTATIONS

1. Start in a high plank position

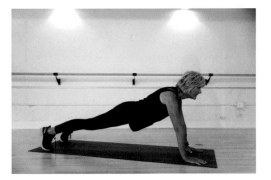

2. Rotate into a high side plank position by rolling onto the sides of your feet and pointing your top hand towards the ceiling so your body resembles a "T"

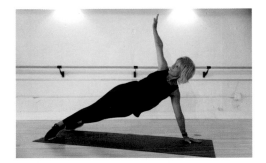

3. Rotate back into the high plank position
4. Rotate into a high side plank position on the other side
5. As you change positions try to keep the same straight alignment from your shoulders to your feet and rotate your hips and shoulders at the same time

TRY THE PLANK PYRAMID CHALLENGE

If you are wanting to get a strong core, then try this tried and true program using planks.

1. Get in a front or high plank position
2. Hold the plank for 10-12 seconds
3. Rest for 5-10 seconds
4. Repeat for a total of 5 planks
5. Rest 1 minute
6. Repeat for a total of 4 planks
7. Rest 1 minute
8. Repeat for a total of 3 planks
9. Rest 1 minute
10. Repeat for a total of 2 planks
11. Rest 1 minute
12. Perform your final plank
13. You're done!!

Advanced Version: Perform the plank pyramid as described above except perform T-Plank Rotations. Hold the initial high plank position for 10-12 seconds before rolling into the high side plank position. Hold that for 10-12 seconds. Roll back into the front high plank position and then roll immediately into a side high plank on the other side. Hold that for 10-12 seconds before rolling back into the high plank position and relaxing. That all counts as 1 plank!

DEAD BUG

1. Lie on your back with knees bent and feet on the floor
2. Point your arms and bent knees to the ceiling so that only your trunk is contact with the floor

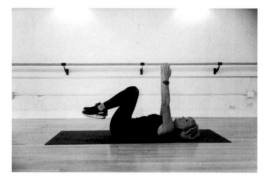

3. Tighten your abdominal muscles before simultaneously extending one arm over your head and straightening the opposite leg

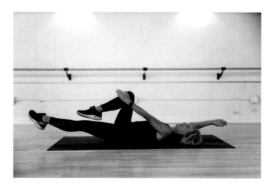

4. Return to the starting position and repeat with the other arm and leg

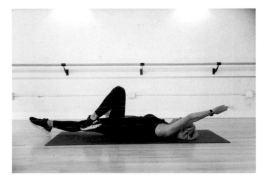

5. During this movement it is important to keep your abdominals engaged so that your back does not arch off of the ground

BIRD DOG

1. Get on your hands and knees with hands directly below your shoulders and knees directly beneath your hips

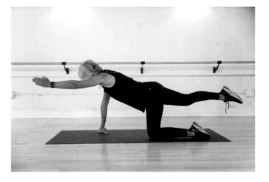

2. Keep your head in alignment with your body so that you are looking straight down at the floor

3. In a slow and controlled manner, extend one arm in front of you (thumb towards ceiling) while simultaneously reaching one leg behind you until they are parallel, or close to parallel, with the floor

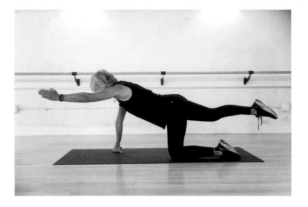

4. Slowly return to the starting position and repeat with the other arm and leg

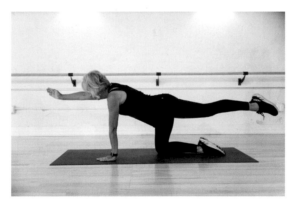

5. Keep your abdominals tight throughout the movement so that your back does not arch, sag or twist. Thinking about reaching your limbs instead of lifting your limbs will help.

Easier Variation for Dead Bug and Bird Dog: Perform either of the movements using only 1 limb at a time. Extend one arm and return to the starting position. Extend the opposite leg and return to the starting position. Repeat with the other arm and leg.

PALLOF PRESS

1. Wrap the tubing around a pole or stair rail and hold both handles together within a clasped fist
2. Turn your body so that the pole is beside you with your elbows bent 90 degrees and pulled tightly into your sides

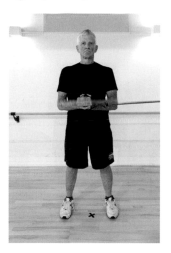

3. Make sure you are in a good upright posture before stepping sideways away from the pole to create tension on the tubing, and assume a shoulder-width stance
4. The tension from the tube will tend to rotate your body so tighten your abdominals and hips to prevent any rotation

5. You can hold this position OR slowly press your hands away from your body (which will make it more difficult) and then slowly return your hands to the starting position before repeating

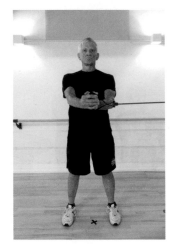

6. Breath shallowly from your upper chest to prevent holding your breath

SNOW ANGELS IN PRONE

1. Lie face-down on the floor (you may place a small towel under your forehead if necessary) with arms stretched overhead

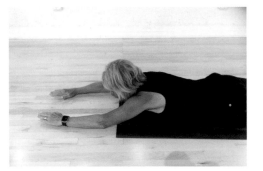

2. Keeping your arms as straight as possible lift your hands off the floor

3. Pull your elbows to your sides without letting them touch the floor

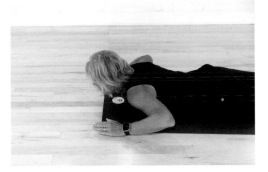

4. Reverse the motion until your arms are once again overhead

SNOW ANGELS IN SUPINE

1. Lie on your back with legs extended and arms stretched overhead

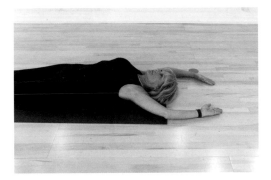

2. Try to contact the ground with as much of your arms as you can

3. Pull your elbows to your sides while maintaining contact with the floor

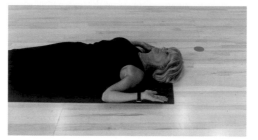

4. Reverse the motion until your arms are once again overhead

The following movements are intended to improve your spinal flexibility, especially in your mid- to upper-back regions, known as your thoracic spine. Having adequate mobility in the thoracic spine is essential to good posture and good movement. Unfortunately, many people lose their thoracic mobility as they get older and do not do anything to maintain it. Poor thoracic mobility can lead to postural issues and shoulder problems and even contribute to falls.

CAT AND COW

1. Start on your hands and knees with hands directly below your shoulders and knees directly beneath your hips
2. Take a deep breath and as you exhale, arch your back to the ceiling (rounding your spine) while dropping your chin to your chest and tucking your hips towards your chest (the "cat" position)

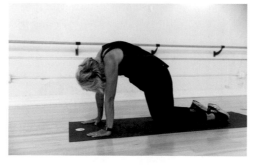

3. As you inhale, reverse the motion to drop your chest and belly towards the floor while looking up at the ceiling and pushing your buttocks towards the back of your head (the "cow" position)

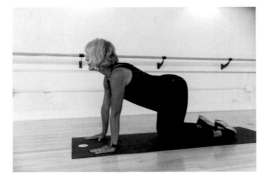

4. Continue cycling through this movement of breathing in and out as you move from cat to cow and back again
5. These should be rather gentle movements so do not try to force your body to move further than it can

EXTENDED CHILD'S POSE

1. Start on your hands and knees with hands directly below your shoulders and knees directly beneath your hips

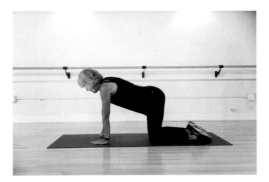

2. Widen your knees a few inches and rotate your feet so that they touch (or almost touch)
3. "Sit" back onto your heels so that your arms are extended
4. Drop your chest between your knees and take your forehead to the floor

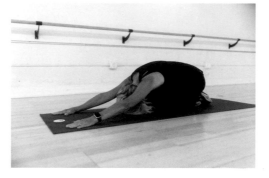

5. In this position, breathe slowly and deeply allowing your chest to sink closer to the floor with each exhale
6. Continue this for 30 seconds

THREAD THE NEEDLE

1. While sitting back in Extended Child's Pose take one arm and "thread" it under the other arm reaching as far as you can so that it twists your upper body

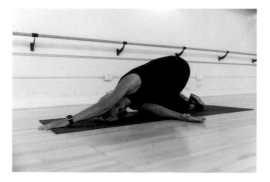

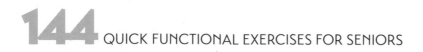

2. Breathe deeply in and out for 30 seconds
3. Reset in Extended Child's Pose and repeat with the other arm

OPEN THE BOOK IN SIDE-LYING

1. Lie on your side with both hips and knees bent to 90 degrees with the top leg stacked on top of the bottom leg
2. Extend your arms in front of your chest with the top arm stacked on top of the bottom arm

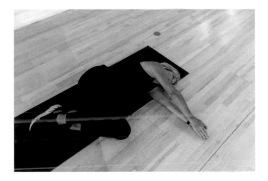

3. It is best to have a small pillow or towel resting under your head
4. Keeping your legs firmly on the floor and stacked together, slowly take your top hand off of the bottom hand by rotating your upper body
5. Try to rotate onto your back to place your top shoulder blade and arm on the floor without changing the position of your stacked legs

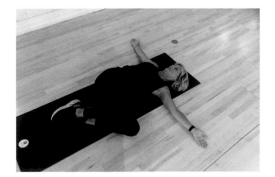

6. The focus should be on your shoulder blade more than on your hand
7. When you have rolled as far as you can go, take several deep breaths. With each exhale try to relax more so that your shoulder blade moves even closer to the floor.
8. Return to the starting position and repeat several times
9. When finished, turn over onto your other side and repeat in the same manner.

CHAPTER 7
Building a Program

Putting together an exercise program may seem daunting at first if you have never done it before, but you will find it isn't quite as difficult as it may appear. It will take a little time to get into the groove of exercising regularly and discovering how your body responds to training. Following are some guidelines to apply when putting together a program along with several example program templates you can use and modify and additional information to guide you in your journey.

SOME BASIC GUIDELINES
1. Remember that almost any kind of exercise is beneficial
There are lots of "right" ways to exercise and many fewer "wrong" ways to exercise. As stated earlier, even the most basic exercise program has lots of value if you do it consistently. It doesn't matter if you go to a gym or work out in your basement or if you use dumbbells or resistance bands. It makes very little difference if you prefer to walk, bike, swim, or row. Therefore, move in ways that are the most enjoyable that will keep you exercising consistently and, when in doubt, just keep moving. At the same time, it is possible that you really don't like any of it or you don't have enough experience to know what you like. In that case, don't let the choices paralyze you. Just choose something and go with it. If you don't like it, then try something else. But don't be too quick to make a judgement.

One of the shows I used to watch was "Bizarre Foods" hosted by Andrew Zimmern. He traveled the world eating the weirdest and often most disgusting foods imaginable. However, no matter how bad the first bite might be, he always took a second. His rule was that you shouldn't judge a food based on the first bite alone and some foods that he didn't like at first, he grew to enjoy over time. That's how I was with coffee. The smell and taste of coffee (no matter how much cream or sugar was in it) was simply gross to me. So, it is interesting that today I am an absolute coffee fanatic. I love good coffee, and the darker and stronger the better (no cream or sugar for me). Exercise is similar. Oftentimes, we don't like something the first few times we do it, but as we get more familiar and comfortable (and often better) at it, we come to "enjoy" it. So, don't be too quick to judge an exercise.

2. To get the best results, prioritize your weakest area(s)

Although following a generic program is good, following an individualized program is much better. You only have so much time and energy to put into an exercise plan and, if you are like me, you would likely get some results quickly. To get the best results, focus on the area(s) that are the worst for you right now. These "weak links" tend to respond rather quickly to training and they are likely holding you back from performing at your best. If you feel like you are really weak, then focus on building strength and power. If you feel like your balance is getting worse, then focus on improving your balance and mobility. And so on. Formal assessments, like the ones included in this book, are one way to identify your weak links. Another way is to think about the types of activities that you struggle with the most. Would being stronger or more powerful help you do them better, or would being more agile on your feet help more?

This is an ongoing process for several reasons. For one, it is too difficult and time-consuming to try to assess every single aspect we've discussed so far. It would take a lot of time and probably some help from an expert. Therefore, follow the principle "the exercise is the test." Every single new movement you try is in and of itself an assessment of your capabilities. It is, therefore, extremely important that you continually introduce new movement challenges into your routine in the different areas we've discussed. You won't know how well or how poorly you can move in specific ways until you try.

Consider the case of my client Bob, a 79-year-old retired pilot preparing to go to Vietnam with his son-in-law and grandson on a 6-day expedition hiking through the world's longest cave system—the Son Doong Cave in Vietnam. Bob was already a relatively fit individual, but he came to me for help because the expedition was going to be strenuous and he wanted to make sure that, being the old guy in the group, he wasn't going to hold them back. Around the third week of training, I asked Bob to perform a "Carioche" (aka Grapevine) movement. For this exercise, you walk sideways by alternating crossing your trailing foot in front of and then behind the lead foot. I explained and then demonstrated this movement for him, but when it was his turn he froze up. After numerous failed attempts I saw that his frustration was building so I moved on to walking with head turns. For this movement, you walk straight ahead but with every step you turn your head to the side of the foot you are stepping with. So you look to the right when you step forward with your right foot and vice versa. You should be able to walk briskly, smoothly, and straight ahead. Again, epic fail. He could not coordinate his head and stepping movements and he was weaving back and forth significantly. The moral of this story is that we never would have known he could not perform these types of movements had he not tried them. Given that he was going to be exploring a cave system, which would require quite a bit of walking, balance, and coordination, while simultaneously wanting to look around at the surrounding beauty, meant this was a skill he needed to master. Again, you won't know if you don't try.

3. Be well-rounded with your time

After first working on your weakest area(s), spend the rest of your time on some of the other areas. Since the law of "use it or lose it" applies to every system in our bodies, we need to challenge as many of them as possible on a regular basis. Don't spend all of your time lifting weights to keep getting stronger and stronger if you are already strong enough but you aren't very coordinated. It would be better to shorten the amount of time devoted to weight-lifting so that you have more time to focus on improving your coordination. This is one of the biggest mistakes I see most older adults make in their programs—being too narrow and focusing on the areas that they are already good at.

If you have more than one area that you have prioritized, then all of your training time may initially be taken up by focusing solely on improving these areas. That's okay for a little while, but eventually you want to include more areas in your weekly program, which might mean that you need to workout on more days per week or workout a little longer each time in order to address them all.

4. Progressive overload

Challenging your abilities is the key to improvement. If a movement is really easy to do, then it likely isn't challenging enough and either needs to be changed or progressed. On the other hand, if you continually try to perform movements way beyond your capabilities, then you will get frustrated or even injured. For example, if you have trouble standing on one leg with your eyes open, then why would you even try to do a backwards tandem walk with your eyes closed? But, if standing on one leg is easy to do, then you need to try something more challenging (closing your eyes, turning your head, etc.). Therefore, always start with something that you think you can be successful with, but once the challenge isn't in the "somewhat hard" to "hard" range, it is time to increase the difficulty level. Don't be surprised when a movement that was quite challenging at first becomes significantly easier after only a short period of time. Some of us adapt more quickly than others.

Typically, a person will have an initial learning period lasting two to three weeks where they are just trying to figure out how to perform the movements appropriately and trying to get in a groove. The next few weeks (eight to twelve or longer) are often followed by some rapid improvement. During this improvement phase, you may find yourself increasing your weights, repetitions, sets, time, number of exercises, etc. on a very regular basis. How exactly you progress each movement depends on what kind of exercise category it falls under. Some ideas for progressions are described later in this chapter. At some point you will settle into a longer-term phase where gains come slower. However, the rate at which you see results and the magnitude of those results are directly attributable to the type of exercise program you are following, your consistency (huge factor), and the effort you are putting into it.

5. Understand the difference between pain and effort

Moving in new and challenging ways will likely be uncomfortable. Sweating, getting out of breath, fatigue, a "burning" sensation in your muscles...these are all to be expected during exercise. Following exercise, you may get sore or feel a little "stiff." At first, these sensations seem to be much worse than they really are because you are not used to them. However, over time, your tolerance will increase and you may even grow to "like" these sensations because you understand that you won't improve without pushing yourself. As someone who has been exercising for almost their entire lives can attest, it gets better. One way to minimize the discomfort is to start at an easy level and progress slowly. Whenever I have had an extended break from exercise I always start back up again at a very, very low level compared to where I was before. Basically, I just go through the motions not even worrying about how much weight I am lifting to give my body (and mind) time to get back into the regularity of training.

Being too aggressive too soon is why the gyms are flooded in January (after the New Year's resolution to lose weight and get in shape) and empty by March. People push themselves too hard too soon. They get overly sore and aggravate their joints and never get into a regular routine.

Also keep in mind that "no pain, no gain" is a half-truth. Effort produces results: TRUE. Exercise should be painful: FALSE. Discomfort due to effort is okay but actual pain, especially in your joints, is not. Do not try to push through your exercise routine when your knees are killing you or you have a really sore muscle or your lower back is hurting. These are all signs that you need to back off, rest/recuperate, or even choose a different exercise. Many exercises can be very therapeutic, but you may have some specific issues that require a more targeted approach than this book can provide. Overall, you should feel better and more invigorated following a training session compared to before your session even though you may also be tired from the effort you just put in.

6. Keys to success

Physical movement, including formal exercise, is such a powerful stimulus for our bodies *if* we are willing to put in the time. The biggest improvements are seen in people who go from doing nothing to doing something, even if they are just following a mediocre program. But as soon as they stop doing it their results quickly diminish. To the contrary, you could have the greatest scientific minds in the world develop the optimal program for you but it won't do you any good if you don't follow the plan. Therefore, the first key to success is consistency. Commit to following the plan each and every day despite whatever else might be going on in your life—travel, special events, holidays, occupational duties, or the dreaded "I'm just not feeling it today." Just show up each and every session you have scheduled. Of course, this means planning ahead and scheduling your sessions into your day just like any other important appointment and then commit to keeping that appointment. Then troubleshoot ahead of time so you don't get in a jam. Going out of town? Where will you exercise? Hotel gym? Local gym? Outdoors? In your hotel room? Do you need to take equipment with you? What if it is too cold or too hot or too rainy? Overcoming situations like these will keep you consistent and will boost your internal commitment. Plus, you will feel really good about yourself. If you are having trouble staying consistent, then consider setting alarms, getting an accountability partner, working out with a spouse or friend, or getting a coach.

The second key to success is effort. Just like anything else in life, you will get out of exercise what you put into it. And for some it might take a great deal of effort to alter their current trajectory and secure a better future for themselves. There will be setbacks and obstacles to overcome. There will be times when you are tired or stressed and you just don't want to push yourself.

The final key to success is positive aging mindset. Mindset is everything. Nelson Mandela is a great example of the power of a positive mindset. Mandela was imprisoned at the age of 44 for his anti-apartheid views and activities, where he remained for 27 years until he was released at the age of 71. During his time in prison, he was regularly harassed by the prison guards and often spent time in solitary confinement. During his incarceration (an 8'x8' concrete cube for a cell), Nelson began an exercise routine that consisted of stationary running, 100 finger push-ups, 200 sit-ups, and other calisthenics, which he performed each morning from Monday through Thursday before resting for 3 days. Once he was released from prison, he took up boxing three evenings a week along with running four mornings a week. He had committed to exercise to not only stay physically fit but to help him endure the mental hardships he faced daily. It would have been so easy for Nelson to get discouraged and depressed for his wrongful imprisonment—to tell himself that he was never going to get out of prison anyway so exercise was of no value. He could have blamed his circumstances, his conditions, or his many obstacles. But he didn't because he had a strong mindset. And that mindset not only kept him physically and mentally fit but garnered him the presidency of South Africa at the age of 76.

With the right mindset you can overcome almost any problem, obstacle, or situation placed before you. However, a poor mindset can sabotage your efforts even before you begin. A positive aging mindset believes:

- You can be fit, healthy, and functional at any age
- Age is not an excuse to be inactive or unhealthy
- Growing older is a badge of honor because it means you have persevered so be proud of yourself
- Most of the "problems" associated with getting older are really due to poor lifestyle choices
- It's never too late to make significant improvements in your health and fitness
- You are only as old as you believe yourself to be

7. Know when you need some help

Recently, our garbage disposal stopped working. I could hear it get power when I flipped the switch, but nothing would happen. I pressed the reset button on the bottom of the disposal. I cleaned it out the best I could to check for anything that might be blocking it from turning. I manually turned the blades using a small wrench (as the instructions indicated). All to no avail. Nothing worked. After fooling with it for a couple of days (trying all of these over and over again), I finally gave in and called the plumber. It ended up the unit was broken and needed to be replaced. There are times when we need to know when to call in the professionals, and exercise programs are no different. Here are some indicators that you need to seek the advice of a fitness professional, wellness coach, physical therapist, or physician.

- Your current conditions get worse, rather than better, with exercise
- You develop new aggravations or problems such as joint or muscle pain that just won't go away
- You injure yourself and aren't sure which exercises you can keep doing and which ones you should avoid for a while
- You do not understand what to do or how to do it by following images or videos of exercise movements
- You cannot maintain consistency due to a lack of motivation or self-discipline
- You are no longer seeing any improvements and aren't sure what to do next to keep getting better

Check out the resources included in this book for even more guidance and assistance to help you be successful in your exercise journey.

PROGRAM IDEAS

There is a lot of helpful information and exercises in this book, but ultimately you have to put pen to paper and actually create an exercise program for yourself. What types of exercises do you do? Which specific exercise movements do you choose? How often do you do them? These are all questions that need to be answered. Below are some example program templates separated into Beginner, Intermediate, and Advanced.

These are just a few of the many ways that you can put together a program and they are generic. You will need to pick a format that works for you and meets your specific needs. If you choose to train a certain area (lower body strength, for example) you want to do so a minimum of 2 days per week. For some areas, much more is recommended.

Cardiovascular exercises can be performed every single day and even multiple times per day, although you will want to alternate between higher and lower/moderate intensity sessions on back to back days unless you are advanced in that area. Strength and power training exercise sessions for a particular part of the body should have 48 to 72 hours of rest between them. If you train the upper body on Monday, you wouldn't want to train the upper body again until Wednesday or Thursday. However, you could easily train the lower body on Tuesday since it is a different part of the body. Core exercises (like planks) can be performed on back-to-back days if you vary the focus of the exercises. For example, if you do front planks on Monday, then do side planks on Tuesday. Posture exercises that focus on mobility and flexibility should be performed as often as possible, as the more you can stretch the better. Balance and mobility exercises can also be performed daily but, like with core exercises, you should change the types of movements on back-to-back days.

BEGINNER PROGRAM

- Walk for 30 minutes 5 to 7 days/week
- Workout 2 days/week for 30 to 45 minutes with 48 to 72 hours between workouts (e.g. Monday and Thursday)
  - Full Body Strength and Power
  - Balance and Mobility
  - Core and Posture

INTERMEDIATE PROGRAM

- Walk for 30 minutes on Tuesday, Thursday, and Saturday
- Workout 3 days/week for 30 to 45 minutes

- Monday and Friday
    - Full Body Strength and Power
    - Balance and Mobility
- Wednesday
    - Core and Posture

ADVANCED PROGRAM I

- Walk/jog/hike for 30 minutes on Wednesday, Saturday, and Sunday
- Workout 4 days/week for 45 to 60 minutes
    - Cardio – HIIT for 20 minutes on Monday and Thursday; Moderate intensity cardio for 30 minutes on Tuesday and Friday
    - Monday and Thursday
        - Lower Body Strength and Power
        - Core and Posture
    - Tuesday and Friday
        - Upper Body Strength and Power
        - Balance and Mobility

ADVANCED PROGRAM II

- Walk/jog for 30 minutes on Saturday and Sunday
- Workout 5 days/week
    - Cardio each day alternating between:
        - 20 minutes HIIT
        - 30 minutes moderate intensity
    - Monday, Wednesday, and Friday
        - Full Body Strength and Power
    - Tuesday and Thursday
        - Balance and Mobility
        - Core and Posture

HOW TO KEEP MAKING PROGRESS

With all types of training, it is important to keep challenging yourself. This can be accomplished in many different ways depending on the type of exercise. Increasing the amount of time (days per week, number of sets, etc.) and intensity are the two basic ways to think about how to progress. Below are some ideas specific to each of the different types of exercises.

CARDIOVASCULAR

- Increase total time to reach 150+ minutes of moderate intensity cardio per week
  - Try to vary the type of cardio (bike, swim, walk/jog, row, etc.)
- Introduce some higher intensity intervals into 2 to 3 sessions each week and decrease total exercise time
  - Note that 1 minute of high-intensity exercise is equal to 2 minutes of moderate-intensity exercise, so still shoot for a total equivalent to 150 minutes of moderate-intensity exercise (e.g. 30-minute high-intensity + 90 min moderate-intensity)

STRENGTH TRAINING

- Start with 1 to 2 sets, eventually increasing to 2 to 3 sets
- Increase load/weight/resistance, so completing 10 to 12 repetitions remains challenging
  - Note: When you increase resistance, your repetitions may drop. Stay at that level until you can complete 12 repetitions for each set several times before increasing the resistance again.
- Move from isolated movements to compound/full-body movements
- Add additional exercises to challenge muscles and movements that need more work or that aren't currently addressed in your program
- Start with 2 days per week and gradually increase to 3 to 4 days per week
  - This will give you more time to work on different muscles and movements so that you continue to make improvements

POWER TRAINING

- Increase your speed until you are moving "as fast as possible"
- For jumping-type movements, stay on the ground at first but move toward leaving the ground
- Change the direction of movement (e.g. front hops to lateral hops)
- Introduce new types of fast movements
- Vary the load/resistance of a movement (remember, you do not have to train heavy)

BALANCE AND MOBILITY

- Narrow base of support
- Add different directions
- Multi-task
- Close eyes
- Increase complexity
- Speed up or slow down depending on the exercise
- Increase time holding a position

CORE AND POSTURE

- For "bracing" type movements (e.g. planks, bird dog, dead bug)
  - Increase sets and repetitions to increase total time holding a position
  - Increase load/weights/resistance
    - Performing a plank with your hands on the floor is much more challenging than a plank with your hands on a bench or countertop
    - Extending your arms and legs longer will increase the challenge of the dead bug and bird dog exercises
  - Increase frequency from 2 to 3 days, or more, per week

- For flexibility/mobility exercises

  - Increase time holding a stretch to reach 30 seconds
  - Increase sets to 2 to 3 for each stretch
  - Increase frequency to 5 to 7 days per week

GET STARTED ASAP

Enough reading. It is time to get started. It has been said that "a journey of 1,000 miles begins with a single step." What will your first step be? Don't overthink it. Don't hesitate. Just act. Overcome your current inertia and just get moving. Remember that movement, and specifically exercise, is powerful. No matter what you choose to do at first, it will be good for you. Don't wait until you think you have developed the optimal program. Don't wait until you have the perfect place to work out. Don't wait until you have all of the equipment you feel that you need. Don't wait for the weather to get warmer or cooler or for your schedule to ease up a bit. The longer you wait, the less likely you will be to start making changes that will impact your today and your tomorrow. It may never be too late to exercise, but the sooner you get started the better.

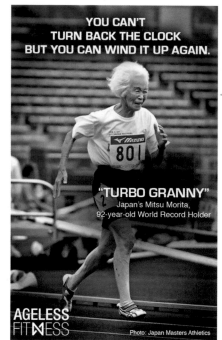

YOU CAN'T
TURN BACK THE CLOCK
BUT YOU CAN WIND IT UP AGAIN.

"TURBO GRANNY"
Japan's Mitsu Morita,
92-year-old World Record Holder

AGELESS
FITNESS

Photo: Japan Masters Athletics

BONUS RESOURCES

Getting started on a new exercise program can be intimidating and I am sure you have lots of questions that weren't answered in this book. I have also found that many people have a difficult time replicating movements from static pictures but do much better with videos. Therefore, I have put together some resources that will add even more value to what you've already received from this book and help you on your journey

FREE ONLINE MEMBERSHIP

Our complimentary online membership site is chock-full of free content and resources to help you on your journey. Simply scan the QR code with your phone (see page 161), or go to the exclusive website link listed at the end of this section, and enter your information to get immediate access. It's that simple. No credit card or payment of any kind is required. This is a gift from me to you to thank you for purchasing this book and to give you the support you need to be successful in your journey toward better health, fitness, and function.

As part of your complimentary membership, you will get access to:

- **The *Quick Functional Exercises for Seniors* Deluxe Movement Library with Videos**
  The online library provides access to images and videos of the exercises included in this book as well as dozens of other exercises that will help you move better and feel better. Zoom in on images to see them better or follow along with the video demonstration so you can better see how it is done from

start to finish. If you have found some of the exercises in this book to be a little too difficult or a little too easy, you will likely find others that better fit your needs and abilities on this site. Want more variety? You will find it here.

- **Follow-Along Brain Fitness Exercise Videos**
  In addition to the numerous bonus functional exercises we have included, you will also get access to follow-along exercise videos to optimize your brain fitness. These are very difficult to do on your own without an instructor so we have put together a series of videos that will lead you through a variety of engaging tasks that will challenge your brain and body simultaneously. Simply play these on your preferred device and follow along.

- **Expert Vault**
  Explore content crafted by a select group of hand-picked experts on topics such as balance, chronic disease, strength, power, longevity, brain health, and more. Get quick tips and pointers to help make your workout even better or dive deeper into a specific topic you are interested in.

- **Exclusive Access to the Members-Only Community on Facebook**
  Need support? Have a question? Want to be motivated and inspired? Have something to share? Our experts and community members are here for you with engaging content, inspiring memes, amazing real-life success stories, and great conversations.

- **Equipment and Product Reviews**
  Find out where to purchase all the equipment listed in this book plus explore many more exercise tools that could be helpful to you. Save time not having to search through Google or Amazon for the right products at the right price because we've done it all for you.

- **Access to Educational Events**
  We will let you know about upcoming webinars, summits, and presentations by internationally renowned experts in their field on topics related to health, fitness, and aging that matter most to you.

To sign up for free, simply scan the QR code at right with your phone or follow this link: www.quickfunctionalexercises forseniors.com/vip

FIND A TRAINER

Are you ready to find a trainer to work with? Maybe you know what to do but have a hard time sticking with it, or you need more help with understanding how to do some of the exercises properly. You may even have some specific physical challenges or limitations that you need to address. Don't worry. We've got you covered. Use the QR code below or follow this link (https://functionalaginginstitute.com/find-a-fai-professional/) to find a qualified fitness

professional in your area. Each of these trainers is a certified Functional Aging Specialist (a certification I personally developed) through the Functional Aging Institute and has completed extensive education on how to train older adults to achieve optimal results. Many hold additional certifications as personal trainers, group exercise instructors, chronic disease specialists, balance specialists, mind-body specialists, and more.

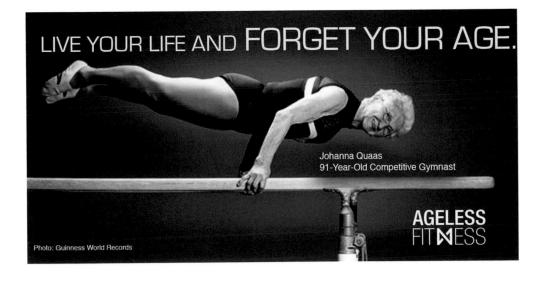

LIVE YOUR LIFE AND **FORGET YOUR AGE.**

Johanna Quaas
91-Year-Old Competitive Gymnast

AGELESS FITNESS

Photo: Guinness World Records

ABOUT OUR MODELS

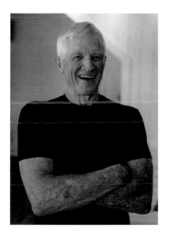

Mike Plummer is a seventy-seven-year-old retired biology professor. As a response to growing up in a largely overweight, sedentary family, Mike vowed never to resort to an unhealthy, sedentary lifestyle. As a result, he has lived an active, outdoor life playing football and baseball through college, semipro baseball in the summers, and, starting at age forty-three, pitching thirty years in the Men's Senior Baseball League. Until Mike had to have both hips replaced at age sixty, he was an avid runner and racquetball player. His most recent passion is pickleball. Mike has maintained his current size and weight since his sophomore year in college.

Jana Adams is seventy-five years old. Having been active her whole life, fitness is very important to her. Currently, her favorite activities are walking with friends, playing pickleball, riding bikes, and hiking. Her main goal is to stay fit and functional as she ages, and staying very active has helped her to do that. She also currently exercises three times per week in a small group personal training program designed specifically for older adults following the functional fitness principles, strategies, and movements found in this book. She now enjoys working on balance, hand-eye coordination, cognitive processing, and explosiveness as well as strength and cardio.

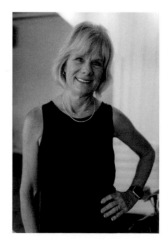

NOTES

NOTES

NOTES

NOTES

NOTES